COPING

WITH

LYME

DISEASE

A Practical Guide to Dealing with Diagnosis and Treatment

DENISE LANG

with Derrick M. DeSilva, Jr., M.D.

An Owl Book
Henry Holt and Company   New York

Henry Holt and Company, Inc.
Publishers since 1866
115 West 18th Street
New York, New York 10011

Henry Holt® is a registered trademark
of Henry Holt and Company, Inc.

Library of Congress Cataloging-in-Publication Data
Lang, Denise V.
Coping with lyme disease: a practical guide to dealing with diagnosis
and treatment/by Denise Lang with Derrick M. DeSilva, Jr.—1st ed.
p.   cm.
"An Owl book."
Includes bibliographical references.
1. Lyme disease—Popular works.
I. DeSilva, Derrick M.   II. Title.
RC155.5L38   1993   93-16442
616.9'2—dc20   CIP
ISBN 0-8050-2650-9

Henry Holt books are available for special promotions
and premiums. For details contact: Director, Special Markets.

FIRST EDITION—1993

Designed by Claire N. Vaccaro

Printed in the United States of America
All first editions are printed on acid-free paper.∞

7   9   10   8   6

FOR CHRISTOPHER,
WHO IS PROVING STRONGER THAN EVEN HE THOUGHT POSSIBLE

Martha Bramhall

Contents

III.
GETTING TREATMENT AND SUPPORT

Acknowledgments

A project as technically and emotionally complex as this book could not have been completed without the assistance of a number of special people. If every cloud has a silver lining, I was granted great riches in the number and quality of folks whose selfless dedication was both an inspiration and tangible help when I needed it.

A debt of gratitude goes to my medical adviser, Dr. Derrick DeSilva, Jr., whose enthusiasm for, and belief in, this book has been matched only by his tireless devotion to educating people about Lyme disease. I am grateful, too, to Dr. John Bleiweiss, Fred Lawson, and Dr. Richard Goldman, who, each in his own way, demonstrate daily a generosity of time and expertise in attempting to relieve the suffering caused by Lyme. And to Dr. Willy Burgdorfer and the scientists of Rocky Mountain Labs, who not only dropped everything to explain the complexities of the Lyme spirochete but were inspirational in their dedication to solving and eradicating the puzzle of Lyme.

Big hugs go to my good friend Ginny Price, who, with sensitivity and conviction, started me on my quest, and to Betty Gross, who pointed out the guideposts along the way and taught me about advocacy. Thank you.

Thank-yous go to the dedicated support group, foundation, and organizational leaders who are touching so many people's lives in a positive way, every day. A number are mentioned by name in the book; most are not. All are thanked.

Special thanks go to my editor, Jo Ann Haun, whose belief not only in the book but in the need for speeding good information to the public has been the force behind this publication; to my research assistant, Kimberly Noon, who jumped in to help with a tight deadline; and to my agent, Martha Millard, whose constant confidence and gentle prodding helped the whole project come together.

Finally, as ever—and especially this time—I owe special thanks to my family: Chris, who traveled the Lyme road to hell and back; Tiffany, who often took a backseat without complaint; and my husband, Larry, who managed, in his steady way, to keep us all on track.

Foreword

Coping with Lyme Disease is a timely book written to help people understand the many confusing aspects of the growing Lyme epidemic in this country and around the world. This book successfully presents and interprets the very complex issues surrounding the disease. Such a book could only have been written by someone who has personally experienced the deep-seated trauma related to Lyme disease within her own family. For the first time, this steadily growing epidemic is presented as a whole picture, and I hope its role as a serious health threat is made more apparent to the general public, physicians, researchers, and government officials.

My career, after pro football, led me to create "The Outdoorsmen," a television show devoted to hunting and fishing. As a result, in 1990 I became interested in learning the facts surrounding a new disease that was alarming the entire outdoor sporting goods industry. Also, at that same time, two of my closest buddies contracted Lyme disease. Both were big, strong outdoorsmen who were literally brought to their knees by Lyme. The pain and suffering associated with the disease incapacitated both of them until each had trouble even lifting a glass of water.

This personal experience left me stunned. As a pro football linebacker for several years with the Los Angeles Rams, I have been blocked by three-hundred-pound offensive linemen with meanness written all over their faces. Sometimes when I got back on my feet it seemed like every part of my body hurt and I would wonder when the stars clouding my vision would disappear. But to witness the enormous pain and suffering caused by a tiny tick no larger than a pinhead is more intimidating to me personally than the meanest offensive lineman I encountered in my entire career.

I am positive the information and knowledge presented in the following pages will help thousands of Lyme disease victims and their families around the world find understanding and proper medical treatment. I am personally asking each of you to share the knowledge you gain from Denise Lang's book with others you know. There are thousands of Lyme victims who every day struggle to have their stories heard. They are the pioneers who have not given up hope their voices will be heard and their prayers answered.

Jim Youngblood, host of "The Outdoorsmen,"
Nord Communications, Greenville, South Carolina

Introduction

The first time I ever heard of Lyme disease was early in 1990, when my five-year-old niece, Lauren, who lives in southern New Jersey, kept falling down.

Her ankles wouldn't hold up this monkey of a child who, uncharacteristically, also complained of headaches, body aches, and joint pain. My sister and brother-in-law made the rounds of doctors (several of whom indifferently said Lauren was just trying to get attention), but it wasn't until she was in such pain that she couldn't get out of bed one morning that someone diagnosed Lyme disease.

We all breathed a sigh of relief. A diagnosis, medicine, a cure, back to good health, life goes on. After all, this is what we are used to and take for granted, we Baby Boomers who have grown up with miracle drugs, immunizations against nature's germs, and high expectations of conquering mountains at a single bound.

I went back to running the treadmill of my busy life: writing books, running a literacy program, trying to keep two teens on track. Long-distance updates on Lauren's Lyme and the doctors who wouldn't officially certify Lyme to the insurance company floated at the perimeters of my consciousness like annoying cobwebs. It bothered me that they were there, but if I didn't look at them, I didn't have to deal with them.

Then one of my most active friends dropped from sight. Linda Martin, professional consultant extraordinaire, talk show favorite, lecturer, etc., etc., was unreachable. The cause? Lyme disease. When I visited her in her upstate New York country house, she was nearly in tears as she told of pain and fatigue so encompassing that she couldn't lift a fork to her mouth. And Linda, who normally speaks at a thousand words a second, carrying on two conversations at once while performing some task, haltingly apologized for not remembering what she had just said.

It affected me. It did. But Lyme disease was still on the perimeter of my life. Again, I was sure that some antibiotic would take care of it and all would go back to normal for her.

So I continued on my breakneck schedule until the winter of 1991–92. And then Lyme disease came into *my* house. It came as a thief, robbing my teenage son first of his health, then of his ability to concentrate and remember, and finally of his dignity and peace of mind. Chris's story is in the chapter on teenagers, but suffice it to say that I became very angry as we fought our way through the medical maze of unknowledgeable diagnoses, insensitive accusations that he must be on drugs (tests proved he wasn't), unenlightened school administrators, and the progressive degeneration of his body while a kaleidoscope of doctors said "Wait and see."

Finally a friend, who had been down a similar road with her daughter, pushed a file folder of information on Lyme disease in my face, and I began to read. As I read, I became even angrier when I realized that Chris had displayed all the classic symptoms and that they had been missed by doctors who didn't put them all together.

By the time I extracted the name of a doctor who specialized in Lyme disease and was put in touch with Derrick DeSilva, Chris was having tremors that lasted hours—and I had decided that Dr. DeSilva was not going to get past me were he to choose not to treat my son. That's how desperate Lyme can make someone who watches a loved one surrender control of not only his body but his spirit as well to a lousy, unseen organism.

Suddenly, Lyme disease wasn't on the perimeter of my life anymore. It was dead center, and it affected how we spent our money, how we spent our leisure time, the tension level in the household, and our views of the future. Not all of our bodies were infected with Lyme, but Lyme had infected all our lives.

And overriding all of this, for me, was anger. Why had the doctors missed obvious signs? Why wasn't the general public more aware of this illness? Why were educators, in whose hands lie our children's self-esteem and future, in the dark? Why were serious consequences denied by the medical establishment? Why was treatment difficult to obtain? And why were insurance companies turning away ill policyholders? The "whys" were deafening.

As a child of the sixties, I am part of the generation that considers it a sacred mission to point to society's ills and try to make changes. Some of my generation have marched in protests. Some have forcibly tried to invade and destroy the establishment. I have used the power of words. But even my years of investigative reporting, writing exposés, and delving into unsavory subjects did not prepare me for the suffering, ignorance, and denial involved in this particular illness.

I've spoken with people across the country who tell stories of medical ignorance and insensitive treatment that contributed to the breakup of families and personalities. I have heard sick children, struggling daily to survive, tell of callousness at the hands of school officials and doctors that would inspire media coverage and protests had it happened to any of our other minority groups. And I've met parents whose highly placed dreams for their children dissolved to longing for simple normalcy, graced by regained health.

I met Polly Murray, the Connecticut mother whose concern over her own children's failing health prompted her to drag Yale

University into the problem, thus "discovering" Lyme disease. I've met a mother whose son, born with congenital problems due to her undiagnosed Lyme during pregnancy, died after living only to kindergarten age. And another mother, whose daughter died of Lyme complications that would not have occurred had her doctors been quicker to diagnose and treat.

I have also talked with people who have given up their life's work to try to educate others on Lyme disease. Those whose dedication and courage have sometimes jeopardized their own livelihoods and reputations. And those who have doggedly pursued an answer to this medical conundrum.

This book is my protest march. I am neither a doctor nor a researcher. I am a mother. I cannot find a cure for disseminated or late-stage Lyme disease. But I can point to the impediments for dealing with this ubiquitous problem facing our environment, our citizens, and our government, and offer some practical steps toward coping with it until the scientists develop reliable tests and solutions.

I hope you will join me. For our families' sakes.

I.

RECOGNIZING THE VARIED ASPECTS OF LYME DISEASE

1.

Lyme Disease: The Cost in Human Terms

"Lyme disease has emerged as a threat to public health worldwide. It is a particularly vexing problem in the United States, where it is growing in range and intensity. In fact, in some regions, it is now such a threat that it interferes with all sorts of outdoor activities and has even led to depreciation of real estate values."

—Dr. Robert Edelman, Professor of Medicine and Associate Director for Clinical Research at the Center for Vaccine Development, University of Maryland School of Medicine

They can tell you to the day—sometimes to the hour—the last time they felt well. These patients who have suffered debilitating symptoms and numerous losses: of jobs, school years, families, relationships, self-esteem, and financial stability. They blame not only the disease but the plethora of doctors who didn't listen, wouldn't believe, or passed them along to other physicians when the diagnosis for this epidemic illness was too challenging. And they are very angry.

The doctors, too, are angry and can't tell you the last time they practiced medicine with the purity and curiosity of spirit inspired by the Hippocratic oath. Some still do, in the face of ridicule from more cynical or sheltered colleagues. And some, who have themselves been victims of this disease—bombarded with tests, interrogations, and skepticism from peers—now view their colleagues in a different light and speak in terms of having to "fight this war" at any cost.

This is the face of Lyme disease.

Once considered only a minor irritation in the northeastern United States, Lyme disease has spread to forty-nine states and eighty countries across six continents, and its pathology embodies some of the medical profession's worst nightmares regarding diagnosis and treatment. The most commonly reported tick-borne systemic illness, Lyme disease has been called the fastest growing epidemic of the twentieth century, second only to AIDS. While, unlike AIDS, Lyme disease is rarely a direct cause of death, misdiagnosis and delay in treatment can lead to permanent disability since the infectious spirochete that causes the disease has an affinity for lodging in, and destroying, major systems of the human body—including the central nervous system, where it evades most antibiotics. It has also been documented as able to hide in the cells and change its presentation, in much the same way as a clever and lethal thief.

Lyme disease is therefore frequently referred to as a disease of morbidity (or sickness) rather than mortality, but it is more than that. If promptly diagnosed and treated aggressively with antibiotics, Lyme disease, theoretically, can be cured, although there is no existing test that will confirm a cured state. However, if, because of its widely confusing symptoms, diagnosis and treatment are delayed, it can become a chronic disease of debilitation—physical, mental, and social debilitation.

So what exactly is the problem? In this age of fast food and modern medical miracles, why can't physicians consider the symptoms, order supportive tests, and begin treatment promptly? The answer promises to inspire a medical Armageddon, so all-encompassing that the legal system, the insurance industry, public health agencies, educational systems, and government entities are all being forced to reevaluate traditionally accepted paradigms.

THE SPREAD OF LYME DISEASE

The story of Lyme disease in the United States began in 1975, when two mothers, alarmed by a rash of cases of joint inflammation in their communities of Lyme and East Haddam, Connecticut, contacted public health authorities. Research scientists at Yale University, headed by Dr. Allen Steere and supported by the National Institute of Arthritis and Musculoskeletal and Skin Diseases, identified what was first known as "Lyme arthritis" in thirty-nine children and twelve adults. Since then, the disease has proven to be more ubiquitous than at first thought.

In 1978 Dr. Steere's team discovered that the disease was being transmitted by the bite of the *Ixodes dammini* tick. In 1981 Dr. Willy Burgdorfer and his colleagues at the Rocky Mountain Laboratories of the National Institute of Allergy and Infectious Diseases, in Hamilton, Montana, isolated corkscrew-shaped bacteria from ticks found in the areas where Lyme disease had occurred. These bacteria were subsequently named *Borrelia burgdorferi.*

The epidemiology of what we call Lyme disease has been traced to the late 1800s, however, and was first described in European literature in 1909 by Dr. Arvid Afzelius, who demonstrated to the Swedish Dermatological Society a migrating annular skin lesion, which he called "erythema migrans" (or EM rash), that had developed at the site of a bite by the sheep tick, *Ixodes ricinus.*

This syndrome and its attendant symptoms have always been referred to in European medical documentation as "Erythema chronicum migrans," or ECM, because of their long duration. It was only in the fall of 1992, when Dr. Burgdorfer, in an attempt to standardize descriptions for a medical profile on the disease, surveyed the international medical community, that all parties agreed to accept the term "Lyme disease."

The Centers for Disease Control (CDC), which is responsible for tracking infectious illness in the United States, has set specific surveillance criteria for reporting purposes that have both allowed public health agencies to follow the spread of the disease and provided grounds for confusion regarding diagnosis (see chapter 6). At the time of this writing, Lyme disease is considered endemic—or regularly occurring—in New York, New Jersey, Connecticut, Massachusetts, Rhode Island, Pennsylvania, Minnesota, Wisconsin, California, and portions of other states, including Georgia, Florida, Louisiana, Texas, and Oregon. As both the public and physicians are educated in recognizing the signs and symptoms of Lyme disease, Missouri, the Carolinas, Alabama, Maryland, Delaware, and a number of midwestern and western states, which are experiencing the spread of the disease, may eventually be added to the list.

As of September 1992, the CDC had recorded 5,485 reportable Lyme disease cases for the year that fit their strict criteria. But—and this is a big "but"—some officials agree that this figure represents only 1 to 20 percent of the actual cases of Lyme, due both to nonreporting on the part of physicians and to the specialized reporting requirements that fit less than 40 percent of Lyme disease cases overall. In some hyperendemic areas, certain communities report that up to 18 percent of the population is infected. Thus, in actuality, the number of Lyme cases for the first nine months of 1992 may be as high as 50,000, and there are many physicians who maintain that the actual numbers are double that. During that same time period, by comparison, reported cases of AIDS totaled 31,455.

These numbers concern not only health officials in the United States but those in the international medical community as well. The spread of Lyme disease has gained epidemic proportions throughout Germany, where an estimated 5 to 10 percent of the entire population is infected, as well as in France, Africa, Australia, portions of China and Japan, twenty-seven Russian territories, and nineteen of twenty-seven European countries.

The big questions regarding the spread of Lyme are how and why and what the government plans to do regarding research funding for a cure.

VECTORS AND HOSTS

In the United States, Lyme disease has been documented as being spread by the *Ixodes* tick. In the North and Southeast it is commonly the *Ixodes scapularis* (formerly called *Ixodes dammini*), and in the West the *Ixodes pacificus*. In addition, there seems to be growing evidence of infection by the Lone Star tick (*Amblyomma americanum*) in the midwestern and western states, and some reporting of infection from the American dog tick (*Dermacentor variabilis*).

In Europe and Asia the predominant vectors, or carriers, of Lyme disease are *Ixodes ricinus* and *Ixodes persulcatus*. There is some controversy both in Europe and in the United States as to whether Lyme is also passed on by other biting insects—such as the mosquito, flea, and horsefly—and some documented cases of this do exist.

These vectors feed on dozens of mammals, birds, and reptiles, which may then serve as reservoirs to infect other ticks. During the tick's three-stage life cycle, it passes from larva to nymph (80 percent of human Lyme disease cases are acquired during this stage) to adult (accounting for the remaining 20 percent). The size of the tick is approximately the size of the period at the end of this sentence.

Despite the fact that the tick must be connected to a human

for at least four to twenty-four hours in order to spread infection, its size, coupled with the fact that it injects an anesthetic into the human skin upon both puncturing and withdrawing, makes it difficult to detect easily.

Although deer and the white-footed mouse have carried the brunt of the blame for spreading the infected ticks, their limited geographic ranges could not account for the rapid spread of the disease. Researchers now agree that infected ticks are hitching rides on ninety-nine different species of migrating birds—and, in fact, tick infestations peak during autumn migration, when an estimated ten billion birds travel up to seven thousand kilometers from summer breeding grounds to winter quarters. During their travels, land birds frequently stop to rest and eat, and they may acquire and pass infected ticks along the way.

In addition, other hosts for infected ticks include more than thirty species of small mammals, including rabbits, voles, chipmunks, and even domestic pets who spend a significant portion of their day out-of-doors. In Europe, additional hosts have included foxes and hedgehogs. And not only can you contract Lyme disease from the infected tick, the disease has been documented in those exposed to the urine or blood of infected animals.

Some researchers maintain that Lyme disease is not necessarily spreading; they say that there is just a greater awareness of it, which has, in turn, caused increasing hysteria, rather than increasing case numbers. This criticism is just wishful thinking. Recent epidemiologic studies find that not only is the tick vector spreading and the percentage of infected ticks increasing, but that such environmental changes as global warming, resulting in warmer winters, have contributed to the lengthened span of the ticks' activity. And despite the indisputable fact that the summer months are prime Lyme season, infection can occur during virtually any month of the year—depending upon one's level of outdoor activity, one's profession, the weather, the geographic location, vacation trips, and whether infected ticks ride into the house on stray mammals (such as mice) seeking warmth during winter months.

Since, at the present time, the most effective weapons against Lyme disease are education and prevention, public health officials, environmentalists, and animal rights advocates are being called upon to assess the efficacy of insecticides and control of the deer population (see chapter 16).

OTHER MEANS OF TRANSMISSION

There is much controversy over the possibility of transmission of Lyme disease by means other than a tick bite. Since the Lyme spirochete, in later stages, has been isolated from various body fluids, there is much discussion regarding the passing of the Lyme infection through blood transfusions, sexual relations, and breast milk.

The Red Cross will not allow anyone who has had an active Lyme disease infection during the preceding year to be a blood donor. Various research studies have shown that the spirochete can live under blood bank conditions for up to several months. In addition, there is a small number of documented cases where a person apparently has been infected through a blood transfusion.

A growing number of doctors agree that, not only can Lyme disease be transmitted through the placenta, but it can also be passed to an infant through breast milk. Again, continuing studies have isolated the spirochete from breast milk and seem to support this position.

One of the more controversial theories is that Lyme can also be transmitted sexually. Although this has not been proven at this time, a number of reputable clinicians maintain that, due to the spirochete's presence in body fluids, the amount of fluid ejaculated during sexual relations would be enough to transmit the spirochete from the male to the female. A number of cases of husband/wife infection have been documented, but further studies have to be undertaken before infection through sexual transmission is proven with any certainty.

THE CONTROVERSIES AND COSTS

"There is no honor in being at the cutting edge of an epidemic."
—Dr. Richard Goldman; Gainesville, Florida; Lyme victim

Darlene is sure she contracted Lyme disease when she was on vacation with her family the year before she entered college. She spent the next four years passing through the revolving door of medical tests, drugs, and increasing symptoms. Her mood swings, fatigue, and varying symptoms cost her a marriage, a job in a brokerage house, and several family relationships. After a suicide attempt, she was assigned to a northeastern psychiatric hospital. When one of the physicians in the hospital, who had been researching Lyme and the illnesses it imitates, initiated Lyme tests for the patients, he was shocked to find that nearly 40 percent of those residing in the psychiatric hospital tested positive. Now, at thirty-four, after six months on intravenous antibiotics, Darlene is just beginning to pick up the life she left behind at eighteen.

■ In today's society, when one feels ill, the course of action is usually quite simple. Depending upon the nature of the symptoms, one might visit a specialist or an internist, who will record the complaints, mentally process the information, issue a diagnosis, and prescribe either a pharmacological remedy or/and a change of habit.

In those cases where symptoms may suggest two or three alternatives, or differential diagnoses, corroborating tests are usually ordered to confirm one or the other, and then a prescription is written. Within a given time period, unless the illness requires surgery or falls into one of the arenas involving AIDS, cancer, or chronic illness, the patient is cured and continues life as before.

Not only have we come to embrace this "cookbook" approach to medical care, doctors themselves are trained to promote it.

Then came Lyme disease. Because of its varied symptoms (many of which are subjective and immeasurable), its varied intensities, its varied stages of development, its ability to masquerade as a number of other illnesses, and the lack of reliable testing procedures for it, Lyme disease has challenged traditional medical practices, polarized the medical community, and raised serious questions regarding health care costs, insurance coverage, and medical malpractice.

It cannot be emphasized enough that Lyme disease, if diagnosed early and treated immediately (defined as within the first six weeks following a tick bite), can usually be resolved without further complications. The problems arise from the following facts:

- More than half of Lyme victims do not remember being bitten by a tick (a tick bite does not hurt due to the anesthetic the tick injects upon both puncturing and withdrawing).
- More than 60 percent of victims do not exhibit a telltale rash (one of the CDC's reportorial requirements—and this includes not just a "classic" bull's-eye rash but ten documented variations).
- The time lapse between the tick bite and emergence of

symptoms can be weeks to months due to the spirochete's slow replication and ability to lie dormant in the human cell, and this can lead to chronic infection.

- Generally accepted testing procedures have had only a 30 to 40 percent reliability rate, at best.
- Too many physicians are ignorant of the disease's complexities at this time.
- Without definitive tests, many physicians have been reluctant to make a diagnosis and begin treatment due to possible malpractice suits.
- Treatment is also a source of disagreement since Lyme does not fit normal patterns of infectious disease containment.

The innate structure of the medical community also lends itself to controversy. There is a traditional dichotomy between basic research (sometimes called "academic" research) and clinical practice.

The researcher wants to control all the variables (as in double-blind studies); therefore subjects are selected, treated, and evaluated uniformly so that scientific principles can be standardized and scientific outcomes can be replicated. The clinician, the "doctor in the trenches" who daily deals closely with suffering people, wants the freedom to treat each patient as an individual, not as a research subject, thus allowing for the very real variations that exist in diagnosis, treatment, and patient response.

Normally, a partnership that meets both sets of needs is forged between the two groups for the overall benefit of science and the patient. But the Lyme spirochete and ensuing infection are proving to be outside the bounds of what has been considered "normal." Therefore, the approach to the disease is going through tremendous "growing pains" even in the heat of battle, complete with verbal missiles launched by both camps of doctors, each with the intention of discrediting the other. Until more time has passed, more documentation has been accepted, more physicians have been educated, more reliable tests have been developed, and more curative antibiotics have been discovered, there will be a difference of opinion and approach.

The media, however well-meaning, have also contributed to the controversy. Whether it is due to lack of space, lack of access to information, or lack of interest in accurately portraying this complex and contradictory medical phenomenon, media coverage has varied from hysterical to myopic to outright denial of the problem.

For example, in the book *Disease Mongers*, author Lynn Payer wrote from a generally confrontational bias against the bombardment of the population by those with a medical agenda to fulfill. She alluded to hysteria over reported Lyme cases and Americans' fear of germs and chose to quote only those few select medical experts who admit to espousing the most conservative (academic) stand regarding Lyme disease despite published documentation to the contrary. This type of one-sided reporting is just as damaging to the education of the public and recognition of a potential health hazard as the denial of the disease's existence and lack of *any* education. Lyme disease, as both researchers and the public are discovering, is not so easily dispensed with in a few simplistic pages.

Finally, there are those self-interested people who are simply out to make a buck off a new phenomenon and who see a new disease as an opportunity for personal and financial advancement. These opportunists can set back the acceptance of well-grounded research and treatment recommendations with tainted practices and attitudes.

But whichever controversy is strongest at the moment, the one who pays the cost is the Lyme disease patient and his or her family, because this is a disease that affects more than just the victim. And the longer the time between tick bite and diagnosis and treatment, the more serious the implications and the higher the costs.

THE APPARENT COSTS

"I scanned my checkbook (can't have a test without a check!) and was able to add up an interesting history before Katie was diagnosed. She saw ten M.D.'s (that we recall) and had three upper endoscopies, one colonoscopy, one lumbar puncture, three upper GI series, one ultrasound, one CAT scan, one MRI, two small bowel series, and blood work done over thirty times (only one was a Lyme titer that I know of). Isn't it unbelievable what our kids have had to endure? The worst part was the lack of understanding and disbelief among the doctors and even our own family!"

—*Liz, registered nurse and mother of teenage Lyme victim;*
Westchester County, New York

In a one-year study conducted jointly by the Society of Actuaries and the Lyme Disease Foundation in 1991 and revised in 1992, the costs of Lyme disease to society were explored. Of the 573 cases originally submitted, the study limited itself to the 503 that reported a documented diagnosis of Lyme disease by a physician.

The study was spearheaded by Dr. Irwin Vanderhoof, an economist and retired adjunct professor at New York University's Stern School of Business, and its results included the following:

- The average number of doctors seen prior to diagnosis was 5.
- A family practitioner diagnosed 146 of the cases; an internist, 96; infectious disease specialist, 85; rheumatologist, 71; neurologist, 70; and other specialists, 69.

- The average lost income before diagnosis was $7,877.
- The average total of medical bills prior to diagnosis was $14,797.
- The average lost income after diagnosis was $6,454.
- The average total of medical bills after diagnosis was $32,560.
- This all came to a grand total of $61,688.
- Further analysis of the data, based on the number of months between the contraction of the disease and its diagnosis, emphasizes the importance of early diagnosis and treatment:

Less than six months until diagnosis—$34,557 average total cost

Seven to twelve months—$68,233 average total cost

Over twelve months—$91,519 average total cost

An examination of individual records determined that 20 percent of the cases—those reporting the largest amounts of cost—represented 80 percent of the total costs. "This is the same relationship we would expect for medical claims in general and those reported to insurance companies," said Dr. Vanderhoof. "The distribution of cost amounts then provides additional credibility to the data. These largest-cost cases averaged thirty-one months from infection to diagnosis and were mostly cases that had some course of treatment with intravenous antibiotics. The average cost reported by these patients was almost $250,000 per case."

Based on the study's overall findings, and taking into account the number of reported and estimated cases, the revised study estimates that Lyme disease costs society approximately $1 billion per year.

Of course, accurate cost determination also goes back to accurate reporting, which concerns the CDC (see chapter 6). Dr.

David Dennis, chief of the CDC's Bacterial Zoonoses Branch and director of its Lyme Disease Program, initiated a survey of fifty-two families throughout five school districts in hyper-endemic New York State in cooperation with the Wharton School of Business to further determine the costs of Lyme.

In addition to the dollar figures, which are consistent with those found by Dr. Vanderhoof, the CDC study also found that among children with Lyme:

- 140 school days were lost, with an average of 98 days of home instruction needed
- 80 percent experienced a drop in grades
- 100 percent had to stop normal social activities
- 80 percent experienced a significant decrease in friendships and other social relationships
- Schools spent $130,000 providing at-home tutoring programs for incapacitated kids
- Total cost per child in the survey, including parents' lost time from work, tests, and treatment, came to $100,000

"Congress allocated $5.4 million for the entire Lyme disease project for 1992–93," said Dennis, "and the actual costs were around $5.2 million for just fifty-two kids. You can see what we're fighting here."

In the employment sector, the costs are also beginning to mount. In those areas where Lyme disease is considered endemic, major employers are not only straining to cover the costs of diagnostic testing and treatment through company benefits programs, but those such as Johnson & Johnson, which self-insures employees, are setting limits as to how much they will pay out.

The 3M Company in Minnesota took a leadership role in educating its population on Lyme by sponsoring a leave of absence for one of its afflicted scientists, Jo Ann Heltzel, with the assignment of researching and teaching the 3M community and its vast environs about the disease—a mission that Heltzel continues.

But aside from the mounting financial costs, the human costs in terms of both adults and children operating at diminished capacity cannot be so easily quantified, and the costs of suffering cannot be translated into dollars.

THE HIDDEN COSTS

At first glance, Sam, a forty-nine-year-old architectural designer, looks like a stereotypical professor or author. Bearded and of robust build, he lived an outdoors life-style on Nantucket with his wife and four children. He traces his Lyme disease to a hike he took in 1987. Through a year of increasing symptoms, beginning with a burning sensation on the bottoms of his feet and progressing to the eventual loss of the use of his legs, he found himself bedridden and dependent, and his symptoms viewed with skepticism. Five years later, he can no longer work at his profession, is divorced, lives in his parents' home, and struggles to simply rise from a chair and move across the room.

"I'm a stubborn Italian and I know I'm going to beat this," he says, "but this disease has cost me in ways you can't even imagine. Your self-esteem drops, you begin to doubt your own sanity, and then you start building walls between you and those around you because they just can't understand what's going on inside. I've always been a positive individual, gregarious, anti-chemical, anti-drug, and now my life has shrunk to just getting through the day. I know what will exacerbate the symptoms, but the limits change each day. What really hurts is what it did to my family," he says softly, eyes filling. "I can't blame my wife. I went through incredible mood swings, hostility, I didn't know what was happening to my body—and since nobody else knew either, no one could tell me, 'Hey, this is part of the disease and you'll get on top of it.' My kids are growing up and I can't be there for them like I'd like to be. I try, but some days are just a struggle to survive the pain. We have to educate not just the people, but the doctors as well. It's better to overdramatize maybe, and save one, than lose many because, man, you lose a whole family—not just a Lyme victim."

■ This story is echoed across the country. Active and upbeat people lose the capacity to perform their jobs; athletes lose their ability to play sports for recreation or profession; the emotional turmoil within family life roils to the point of divorce or separation as the Lyme victim—and in many families, more than one person is afflicted—stresses the climate of a household with constant symptoms, financial demands, and psychological changes (see chapter 5) that boomerang throughout both immediate family and extended relationships.

Because Lyme symptoms can include confusion, short-term memory loss, and disorientation, Lyme victims report withdrawal from not only social situations but also from driving automobiles, for fear of accidents, and from professional situations that might require them to speak before groups or take responsibility for others.

But the losses are even more insidious than that. Since recent studies show that 50 percent of Lyme victims are under the age of twelve, late diagnosis and treatment can result in a potential loss of thinkers, leaders, athletes, dancers, artists, and service providers. In short, the disease is invading the fabric of America's future.

Even the conservative Educational Testing Service in Princeton, New Jersey, which has responsibility for the administering and grading of the SAT, has recognized the effect of Lyme disease on teenagers by implementing a special untimed test for those who can document the illness through a physician. And university admissions offices are becoming increasingly aware of the drop in performance during the high school years caused by Lyme and are accepting students who, again, provide adequate documentation.

Dr. Joseph Burrascano, a nationally recognized Lyme researcher and clinician, who contracted the disease when he was in his teens, says that one's level of performance and expectations are lowered. "Most of the time I felt lousy and I was sleeping sixteen hours a day, but that was normal for me. I didn't realize that other people didn't feel that way."

Lyme disease is changing the way many Americans are spending their leisure time. This includes eliminating nature walks and picnics, not playing in or raking fall leaves, and avoiding contact with certain family pets like dogs and cats in endemic areas. Schools are eliminating recreational and natural-science field trips and there are reports of summer camps closing in endemic areas.

Another real factor in Lyme disease is fear. Some say this is related to modern man's primal fear of the wilderness. But others contend that it is more anxiety and frustration at being attacked in one's own home, or "castle." Dr. Len Sigal, chief of rheumatology and director of the Lyme Disease Unit at Robert Wood Johnson Medical Center in New Brunswick, New Jersey, who cautions against the possible hysteria of seeing Lyme under every leaf, nevertheless understands the public's anxiety. "I moved out of the city so my children can grow up not getting mugged and breathing clean air. Now there's a silent and unseen danger lurking right out in our back yards. This is frustrating."

My grandmother, who seemingly had an adage for everything, loved to repeat that favorite "If you have your health, you have everything." For growing numbers of Lyme disease patients, the "everything" is elusive, resulting in the mental jump to "I have nothing." This is not true. These people have a will to survive, to fight, and to reclaim the good health they wistfully remember. The irony of Lyme disease is that anyone else fighting for health finds a pyramid of support, beginning with physicians and followed by larger tiers of associations, friends, and family.

Lyme disease victims, however, often find themselves stranded on the peak of the pyramid all alone, fighting for credibility, treatment, and simple compassion. Since the symptoms and signs are so varied and often transient, the patient needs to be vigilant in noticing and reporting these bodily and personality changes, and then in seeking the right doctor to put them all together.

2.
Recognizing Symptoms and Seeking Help

When my son was becoming progressively more ill, prior to his Lyme diagnosis, the wide variety of his symptoms seemed staggering; his complaints were constant and every system of his body was involved. In fact, it got to the point where I wondered if he could possibly be making them up, and he wondered if he should even tell me everything that was going on.

As both his body and his personality continued a marked deterioration, however, it became apparent that something serious was definitely wrong. It wasn't until a good friend, who had traveled a similar road the prior year with her daughter, handed me some information on Lyme disease that I began to put the myriad symptoms into a definable context. The turning point was Dr. Burrascano's page of Lyme disease symptoms. In reading this and checking off what Chris had experienced, I realized that this child had thirty out of the forty symptoms listed! He was not a hypochondriac or going crazy, although he was sure he was headed in that direction.

That was two years ago. At that time, doctors dealing with Lyme disease divided it into early and late stages, depending upon the various manifestations of the infection. Since that time it has further been divided into three stages, as doctors and researchers gradually learn more and narrow down the disease's progress. But the doctors emphasize that these stages can overlap—due to individual body chemistry, one person can go from early (which is simply defined as evidence of EM rash) to late disseminated (where the infection has spread throughout many body systems) or even to chronic within months, while another will take months just to go from early to early disseminated.

For this reason, and for clarity's sake, I am going to ignore the stages breakdown at this time and simply present symptoms as they are known today. We will deal with stages in chapter 12.

In an attempt to document as complete a list of symptoms as possible, Kathy Cavert, a registered nurse from Independence, Missouri, editor of *LymeAid* and head of the Midwest Lyme Disease Association, composed a questionnaire and distributed it to more than one thousand Lyme disease patients. In presenting the following list of symptoms, I have combined Dr. Burrascano's original list with the format and additions of Cavert's.

LYME DISEASE SYMPTOMS

As part of your current illness, have you had any of the following?

■The Tick Bite

1.	Tick bite (deer, dog, or other)	Yes	No
2.	Rash at site of bite	Yes	No
3.	Rashes on other parts of your body	Yes	No
4.	Rash basically circular and spreading out	Yes	No
5.	Raised rash, disappearing and returning	Yes	No

■Head, Face, Neck

6.	Unexplained hair loss	Yes	No
7.	Headache, mild or severe	Yes	No
8.	Twitching of facial or other muscles	Yes	No
9.	Facial paralysis (Bell's palsy)	Yes	No
10.	Tingling of nose, cheek, or face	Yes	No
11.	Stiff or painful neck	Yes	No
12.	Jaw pain or stiffness	Yes	No
13.	Sore throat	Yes	No

■Eyes/Vision

14.	Double or blurry vision	Yes	No
15.	Increased floating spots	Yes	No
16.	Pain in eyes, or swelling around eyes	Yes	No
17.	Oversensitivity to light	Yes	No
18.	Flashing lights	Yes	No

■Ears/Hearing

19.	Decreased hearing in one or both ears	Yes	No
20.	Buzzing in ears	Yes	No
21.	Pain in ears	Yes	No
22.	Ringing in one or both ears	Yes	No

■Digestive and Excretory Systems

23.	Diarrhea	Yes	No
24.	Constipation	Yes	No
25.	Irritable bladder (trouble starting, stopping)	Yes	No
26.	Upset stomach (nausea or pain)	Yes	No

■Musculoskeletal System

27.	Joint pain or swelling	Yes	No
28.	Stiffness of joints, back, neck	Yes	No
29.	Muscle pain or cramps	Yes	No

■Respiratory and Circulatory Systems

30.	Shortness of breath, cough	Yes	No
31.	Chest pain or rib soreness	Yes	No
32.	Night sweats or unexplained chills	Yes	No
33.	Heart palpitations or extra beats	Yes	No
34.	Heart blockage	Yes	No

■Neurologic System

35.	Tremors or unexplained shaking	Yes	No
36.	Burning or stabbing sensations in the body	Yes	No
37.	Weakness or partial paralysis	Yes	No
38.	Pressure in head	Yes	No
39.	Numbness in body, tingling, pinpricks	Yes	No
40.	Poor balance, dizziness, difficulty walking	Yes	No
41.	Increased motion sickness	Yes	No
42.	Lightheadedness, wooziness	Yes	No

■Psychological Well-being

43.	Mood swings, irritability	Yes	No
44.	Unusual depression	Yes	No

45. Disorientation (getting or
    feeling lost)   Yes   No
46. Feeling as if you are losing
    your mind   Yes   No
47. Overemotional reactions,
    crying easily   Yes   No
48. Too much sleep, or insomnia   Yes   No
49. Difficulty falling or staying
    asleep   Yes   No

■Mental Capability

50. Memory loss (short or long
    term)   Yes   No
51. Confusion, difficulty in thinking   Yes   No
52. Difficulty with concentration or
    reading   Yes   No
53. Going to the wrong place   Yes   No
54. Speech difficulty (slurred or
    slow)   Yes   No
55. Stammering speech   Yes   No
56. Forgetting how to perform
    simple tasks   Yes   No

■Reproduction and Sexuality

57. Loss of sex drive   Yes   No
58. Sexual dysfunction   Yes   No
    Females only:
59. Unexplained menstrual pain,
    irregularity   Yes   No
60. Unexplained breast pain,
    discharge   Yes   No
    Males only:
61. Testicular or pelvic pain   Yes   No

■General Well-being

62.	Unexplained weight gain, loss	Yes	No
63.	Extreme fatigue	Yes	No
64.	Swollen glands	Yes	No
65.	Unexplained fevers (high or low grade)	Yes	No
66.	Continual infections (sinus, kidney, eye, etc.)	Yes	No
67.	Symptoms seem to change, come and go	Yes	No
68.	Pain migrates (moves) to different body parts	Yes	No
69.	Early on, experienced a "flu-like" illness, after which you have not since felt well	Yes	No

As you can see, this is a daunting list of possible symptoms, but answering yes to many in various systemic categories should put both you and your doctor on the alert to consider Lyme disease. As many doctors who treat Lyme patients say, at one time or another most of us will experience illness in one of our body's systems. If a person is unlucky, he or she can have two major systems involved. But when you begin having problems with multiple systems in the body, that is a red flag to consider a multisystemic infection like Lyme disease. This suspicion should be particularly warranted if you live in an area where Lyme is endemic.

One of the more frightening aspects of Lyme is that, unlike other purely systemic illnesses, it attacks not only the physical well-being of a person but the emotional and psychological components as well. Primary among these symptoms are the mood swings, memory loss, and confusion that Lyme sufferers experience.

Dr. John Bleiweiss is an internist in Trenton, New Jersey, who has been treating (and documenting) Lyme patients with a combination of aggressive therapy and nutrition since 1987. A member of the medical advisory board for the Prevent Lyme Foundation, he has personally struggled with Lyme disease for years and has seen it touch his family. He bristles at the doctors who dismiss the disease as a minor irritation.

"This is the kind of disease which, if not recognized and treated promptly and completely, can affect the future of our country," said Bleiweiss. "I have seen active, outgoing people wind up in wheelchairs without the proper treatment. Nearly all patients complain of 'foggy brain' or 'Lyme fog,' forgetfulness, anxiety, and confusion or disorientation when attempting intellectual tasks.

"Short-term memory impairment causes patients to forget why they entered a room; forget the previous sentence or paragraph while reading; forget dates, schedules, where objects were placed, and even the names of family members. A mother with Lyme left her infant and baby carriage in my parking lot and went home. One patient wandered around the room looking for the pencil that was clenched in his teeth. One patient drove to Philadelphia by mistake instead of Princeton because both began with the letter *P*. In fact, patients can lose their way home, their way to work, or even the way to their classroom in a familiar school because they suddenly forget where they are," he said. "This is scary stuff. And when you think that more than fifty percent of those infected with Lyme disease are teenagers and kids, we're talking about a real impact on our future."

Since the symptoms of Lyme disease are so diverse and progressive, remembering them may be a chore in itself in presenting an accurate accounting to a doctor. The best method to employ is to write it all down.

KEEP A JOURNAL

Like most outdoors enthusiasts, Caitlin had her share of bug bites and rashes. An artist, aerobics instructor, and dedicated hiker and camper, she tried to live a healthful life-style and had little contact with doctors. Then she went hiking in the hills of upstate New York and her life changed irrevocably.

It began with a raised rash, warm to the touch. Since it was unusual, she made an appointment with her doctor. By the time of her appointment to see him two days later (rashes, she was told, are not priority cases) the rash had disappeared, so she canceled the appointment. Then came the headaches and stiff neck. Since she is active, she suspected that she had either overextended herself or slept wrong. When she began to lose the use of her right arm and hand, she went to see a neurologist, and one CAT scan, MRI, and spinal tap later, was told there was nothing wrong with her. The neurologist suggested that perhaps she just needed to take a break from her normal routine. Feeling confused, she ignored the sore throat, the change in bowel habits, and the increasing fatigue she felt. When she found that she was so dizzy she could barely walk, and her arm was so useless that she could not hold her toothbrush, she went to an internist, who ran another battery of tests, told her they were negative, and recommended she consider seeing a psychiatrist since, after all, she was twenty-eight years old and didn't have a steady boy-friend.

"I was so mad, that's when I began writing all the symptoms down," she said. "After a while, I began to think I was going crazy, since every day brought more aches and pains. I had to stop teaching aerobics, I could barely hold a paintbrush, and I was so depressed I didn't even want to be around people. When my mother called to ask how I was, I lied so I wouldn't sound like a hypochondriac and worry her."

Then she passed out in a grocery store and awoke in the hospital, connected to a heart monitor. A cardiologist told her that she had some extra heartbeats and she needed to take it easy and live a more healthful life-style. She never saw him after that. Six months later, Caitlin saw a television program on Lyme disease. A lot of what was being said began ringing bells in her head and she looked at her list of symptoms. She could track the deterioration of her health back to those fateful rashes. A visit to a local Lyme support group meeting put her in touch with a doctor who had experience in diagnosing and treating cases. Her symptom log assisted in his diagnosis.

Eighteen months after Caitlin saw the rash, she is on antibiotics and is beginning to experience a few pain-free days. "But my joints and back still hurt and I find I get lost sometimes. When that happens I just have to calm myself down and keep driving until something looks familiar again," she said with a sigh. "I have to think that someone will come up with a cure someday because there were so many things I wanted to do in life. Now I'm happy just to have a day where I don't drop things, don't have headaches, and can sleep through the night like a normal person."

Caitlin's case illustrates a couple of interesting points. First, by the time she could get a doctor's appointment, her rash was gone. Therefore, there was no documentation of the rash—the first criterion for reporting Lyme disease—by a physician. Second, Caitlin, accustomed to thinking in terms of medical specialties, in her attempt to get a diagnosis from her symptoms saw several different types of doctors, each of them only seeing what applied to his or her area of expertise. This is very common. It was only due to Caitlin's efficiency in writing down her symptoms that her physician was able to piece together a difficult diagnosis.

As information regarding Lyme disease spreads throughout

the country, perhaps doctors will make room for patients who call complaining of suspicious rashes. Until then, I would encourage anyone with a suspicious rash to go to one of the fine walk-in emergency medical centers popping up across the country. No appointment is necessary, and if the rash turns out to be the hallmark of Lyme, you will have a doctor's confirmation of its presence.

Dr. Ernest Biczak trained in emergency medicine as preparation for opening his Immediate Medical Care Center in rural Chester, New Jersey. "Eleven years ago when we opened, I thought we would be handling emergencies, but what we've turned into is a family practice," he chuckles. "This is what has been the greatest need in our area. And we've been seeing more Lyme rashes this year than ever before. Some days, we will get three in a single day. Other days, none. We have talked about bringing in a camera to photograph and document them and we may have to do that yet."

Since contracting Lyme disease begins with a very specific event—the bite of a tick—it presents a very definite onset of symptoms. Whether you remember a tick bite and rash, or fall into the 50 percent who don't, when experiencing vague, fluctuating, or increasingly disturbing symptoms, it would be a good idea to take the time to write them all down in a time-line fashion to the best of your ability. Get a family member to help you, if you can't remember. Do not leave anything out—from mood swings to weakness in a particular extremity.

This symptom log or journal can be a simple listing of symptoms; you do not need to write long paragraphs. Some doctors advise their patients to include a "wellness indicator" as you are going through the testing and diagnosis process. This is simply a scale from 1 to 10, with 10 for feeling great and 1 for feeling the worst. Assign a number to each day to aid the documentation of progress or degeneration. This will assist doctors as they consider various diagnoses.

THE DIFFERENTIAL DIAGNOSES

Jo Ann was diagnosed as having multiple sclerosis. After six years of treatment for MS, with continual degeneration, she was tested for Lyme and found to have the disease. Treated with antibiotics, she began to recover her physical and mental abilities, her job performance, and her life. Today she is working to educate others regarding Lyme disease and includes the warning that it masquerades as many other illnesses, not the least of which is MS.

Twelve-year-old Dennis was told he had chronic mononucleosis and attention deficit disorder (ADD). As he deteriorated from a normal, active adolescent with hopes and dreams to sitting in a wheelchair and being assigned to a special education class, his parents struggled for help. He was finally tested for Lyme, in spite of opposition from his pediatrician. After nine months of therapy, Dennis is finally rejoining his classmates in thinking about high school next year and trying out for sports teams.

Beverly felt her life was over when her doctor told her she had lupus. It was only after two years of meticulous research on the part of her husband and a change of doctors that she was tested for Lyme disease. Since she lives in Texas, an area where Lyme disease supposedly does not exist, she travels to California for treatments. It is a small price to pay, she says, for feeling better and getting back her life.

■ Lyme disease is a clinical diagnosis and may become a diagnosis of exclusion. This means that, unless you exhibit a classic rash and test positive by blood, the physician will attempt to eliminate all other possible diseases before making the Lyme diagnosis. This is not unreasonable. Called the "New Great Imitator," Lyme disease, because of its myriad symptoms, can mimic two hundred other illnesses. As a result, it can be missed by doctors who are not well acquainted with its pathology and progress.

There are several diseases that Lyme mimics most frequently, and, in discussing Lyme with your doctor, he may give you a "differential" or alternate diagnosis as you go through the testing process. These include:

Multiple sclerosis   A chronic, demyelinating central nervous system disease, similar to Lyme. Recent medical literature has drawn parallels between the two diseases in that magnetic resonance imaging (MRI) tests cannot distinguish between Lyme and MS; spirochetes have also been found in the spinal fluid and tissue samples of MS patients; and great clusters of MS victims have appeared in those areas of the United States and around the world where Lyme is now endemic. Some researchers are studying whether the Lyme spirochete, in fact, could be one of the causes of MS or if the Lyme spirochete produces the MS-like, Lyme-like illness.

Fibromyalgia   An inflammation of the connective tissues of the body. It is a chronic pain syndrome characterized by diffuse muscle and joint pain; headache; abnormal spontaneous sensations such as burning, pricking, and numbness; sleep disturbances; and fatigue. Symmetric tender points are usually found in various locations over the neck, back, and extremities. Women are affected more frequently than men, with no apparent explanation.

Systemic lupus   A disease characterized by inflammation in many different systems. Patients may have fatigue, anemia, fever, rashes, sun sensitivity, arthritis, pleurisy, hair loss, and nervous system disease. This disease, like Lyme, waxes and wanes in intensity, and its hallmark is a distinctive "butterfly" rash across the face.

Infectious mononucleosis   An acute infection caused by the Epstein-Barr virus. Symptoms include fever, sore throat, swollen glands, and fatigue. When confronted with confusing symptoms, some doctors have diagnosed chronic mono, but many more debate its existence, labeling it a "catchall" diagnosis.

Amyotrophic lateral sclerosis (ALS)   Also known as Lou Gehrig's disease, it affects the muscles in a single limb or all four limbs simultaneously and runs a course from two to seven years. A fatal disease, it usually strikes those in their fifties to seventies. Despite extensive research, the cause of ALS remains unknown at this time.

Chronic fatigue syndrome (CFS)   This disease, also referred to as the Yuppie disease, is caused by a virus and therefore does not respond to antibiotic treatment. Since severe fatigue—in fact, chronic fatigue—is a hallmark of Lyme disease, there are many doctors who insist that many Lyme patients are being misdiagnosed without being given a chance to be treated. Five million people have been diagnosed with CFS, yet the diagnosis is confusing, says Joe Burke, founder of the American Lyme Disease Alliance and formerly diagnosed with CFS. "A lot of the people who go to chronic fatigue support groups are also Lyme disease patients; many more exhibit classic Lyme symptoms but won't even seek a Lyme test or diagnosis because having CFS is a more comfortable plateau than looking further."

Alzheimer's disease   This most common of the progressive dementias affects both men and women. It primarily strikes the elderly and can exhibit many of the symptoms of Lyme, especially those of a cognitive nature; therefore a particular danger of misdiagnosis exists when dealing with senior citizens (see chapter 10).

■ Another roadblock to the accurate diagnosis of Lyme is the type of doctor you seek out. Because Lyme affects many systems of the body, a specialist for one system may not be able to look at the total picture of symptomology and make the diagnosis.

For example, the neurologist will consider the headaches but not the heart palpitations or joint pain. The rheumatologist will focus on the joint pain and the immune system but will probably pay little attention to the deterioration of your eyesight that is going on concurrently, referring you to an ophthalmologist . . . and so on.

Your primary line of attack should be an internist or family medicine practitioner, who should begin with a thorough patient history, some basic tests, and then coordinate with other specialists as needed. You need someone who can look at the overall picture and put the puzzle of Lyme disease together.

This, of course, assumes that the doctor you see is willing to work with you to find the right diagnosis. The key words here are "work with you."

THE VOLATILE DOCTOR-PATIENT RELATIONSHIP

When Lauren was five, she was diagnosed with Lyme disease after eleven months of misdiagnoses. Treated for three months, she seemed relieved of all symptoms and continued with life. When she was eight years old, her symptoms seemed to be returning. Back again were the joint pains, the headaches, and the stomachaches, plus—a new wrinkle—pain in her chest.

Her mother, taking her to a new pediatrician (her old one had retired), mentioned that Lauren had previously suffered from Lyme and had responded to treatment. In view of the recent medical literature indicating that the spirochete can lie dormant in the body for years and then flare up, she wanted the doctor to know her daughter's background. Since they live in one of the most highly endemic areas of Lyme disease in New Jersey, she felt this information would be pertinent in case the chest pains and other symptoms were part of the old disease rather than a new one.

"The doctor went crazy," said the stunned mother. "He actually screamed at me that Lyme disease was being blown out of proportion by hysterical women and irreputable doctors. He accused me of looking for Lyme under every symptom, and blasted me for mentioning the recent articles on Lyme, saying, 'And just where does one go to be an expert in Lyme disease, huh? Are there schools that teach Lyme disease?' He refused to examine my daughter that day—said he didn't have enough time because he had 'really sick patients to see' and that I could make another appointment if I felt it was really necessary.

"I can't believe he treated us that way. He refused to see a child who was complaining of chest pain and went nuts on me, all because I was trying to give him an accurate background to evaluate my daughter. Believe me, I am not an hysteric, but that doctor is also not a responsible physician! I wonder how many kids in this area are sick with Lyme because he refuses to even consider it when examining his patients!"

■ Approximately sixteen thousand new doctors graduate from this country's 128 medical schools each year. Somewhere between internship and residency, unfortunately, many new doctors tend to develop an arrogance that goes beyond the confidence one must have in order to make life-and-death decisions for another human being. While this arrogance is variously tolerated by Baby Boomers and expected by senior citizens, it can serve as an obstacle to good care.

Unfortunately, too, this arrogance is encouraged by the very people it can hurt. In this age of medical miracles, when we expect quick cures to difficult problems, the physician is trained to come up with those answers and cures. In fact, he is trained to come up with something—anything—when the patient asks a question; for to say "I don't know" is viewed as the ultimate sin.

There is a lot that scientists, researchers, and doctors admit they don't know about Lyme disease. Worse yet, there is much that is known and ignored in medical teachings and practice. Those who make that admission and proceed from there are light-years ahead of those who deny the ubiquitous and diffuse nature of the illness because they are threatened by not having the answers.

There are two cardinal rules in coping with Lyme or suspected Lyme disease:

1. Do not accept ignorance or arrogance from your doctor.
2. Take an advocate with you to your medical appointments.

DO NOT ACCEPT IGNORANCE OR ARROGANCE FROM YOUR DOCTOR

When you take your car in for repair, you expect the mechanic to listen to your list of complaints, make his own observations, and then attempt to fix your car. If you get that car back, but it is still rattling at fifty miles per hour, you would probably return it to the mechanic and point out the problem. You would, rightly, expect him to work on it again to find out what the cause of the rattle could be.

If, however, the mechanic told you that the rattle was all in your head, belittled your intelligence, cross-examined you, and stated that if he said it was fixed, then it was fixed, would you go back to him? Of course not.

Yet many of us don't give our bodies and our health the same respect that we give our cars. The mechanic may know more about cars, but it does not follow that you cannot make valid observations.

By the same token, when confronted by a doctor who does not listen, will not take the time to ask questions of you, is threatened by your questions or information, and tells you that "she" is the doctor and "you" are the patient, and therefore know little about medicine, you must fire her and search for a doctor who will work with you.

Alfred Adler, often referred to as the father of individual (termed Adlerian) psychology, wrote about the arrogance of doctors back in the 1930s. He said: "To be a physician may mean many things. Not only may he wish to be a specialist . . . but he will show in his activities his own peculiar degree of interest in himself and interest in others. We shall see how far he trains himself to be of help to his fellows and how far he limits his helpfulness. He has made this his aim as a compensation for a specific feeling of inferiority; and we must be able to guess, from his expressions in his profession and elsewhere, the specific feeling for which he is compensating."

Any doctor who is threatened by a reasonably questioning patient is not someone you can trust to work with you.

It is equally unproductive, however, for a patient to walk into a doctor's office, present a list of symptoms, a diagnosis, and demand therapy of a specific sort. Confronted with that kind of patient, more often than not, a doctor could reasonably say, "Why do you need me if you have all the answers?"

TAKE AN ADVOCATE

Anyone who has received either shocking or complicated medical information knows that the mind tends to block the flow of information with emotional linebackers. Afterward, you might wonder, "What did the doctor say again?"

Since short-term memory loss, confusion, and fatigue are definite hallmarks of Lyme, it is a particular advantage to have a relative or other advocate present to absorb the doctor's spoken information, assist in remembering symptoms and events, and help with recommended tests or therapies.

Most children have a built-in advocate in Mom or Dad— whoever is the primary parent taking them through the sick-to-well process. But sick adults—particularly those who suspect Lyme—need an advocate as well.

Even in the best of circumstances, when one is ill it is difficult to remember all that the doctor has said and recommended. A discussion of Lyme disease can provoke anxiety that causes the patient's memory to go blank, and it helps to have another pair of eyes and ears and another brain to absorb, remember, and ask the right questions.

As we hurtle into the twenty-first century with its complex diseases and life-styles, a new type of doctor-patient relationship must be forged: a partnership whereby the doctor and the patient (the medical consumer) work together to seek resolution of a medical problem. We must work toward a "therapeutic alliance."

3.
Developing a Therapeutic Alliance

"Kinship is healing; we are physicians to each other."

—Oliver Sacks, *Awakenings*

During the mid-1800s, the Countess Rosa Branka, of Poland, upon being diagnosed as having breast cancer, decided to take matters into her own hands—literally. Distrustful of the doctors, she amassed surgical instruments and performed surgery on herself, excising the cancerous lump. She lived another twenty-one years in good health.

While not many people would resort to the countess's drastic measures, the relationship between doctors and patients can be strained to the breaking point at a time when the two should work closely together. As one mother of a Lyme sufferer said: "The easy stuff they can treat. It's how they handle the difficult illnesses that lets you know the kind of doctor you have. This is when you get to see the heart and soul and guts of your doctor."

In approaching Lyme disease, as with any complicated illness, the doctor needs to throw away the "medical cookbook" and get to work as a detective, piecing together the clues to the final diagnosis. This may require a change of practice and attitude, not only among the doctors involved but for the patients as well.

In speaking with both physicians and Lyme patients across the country, I have been able to categorize the ways in which a good working relationship can be sabotaged.

HOW PATIENTS OBSTRUCT THE DOCTOR-PATIENT RELATIONSHIP

1. The "It's my doctor's job to keep me well" attitude.

This type of attitude leads patients to abdicate responsibility for good health practices. It allows them to smoke, drink to excess, and ignore good dietary recommendations, thereby sabotaging both antibiotic treatment and the immune system.

As medical consumers—and we must begin to think of ourselves that way—it is *our* job to keep ourselves well; it is the doctor's job to find out what is wrong when we are unwell and make *recommendations* to "fix" us.

2. Diagnosing oneself and demanding specific therapy.

Since, to this point, the medical profession as a whole has not been well informed regarding Lyme disease, this is a very real pitfall when a patient is seeking diagnosis. There is no doubt that many patients have been better informed than their doctors regarding this disease. By the same token, the doctor must have a healthy skepticism and eliminate other possibilities as well. If you find a doctor who is informed on Lyme, let him do the job he was trained to do. Remember, other diseases must be ruled out.

3. Concealing important information.

There are patients who will say only what they think the doctor wants to hear, whether to save embarrassment, to cover up some "health sin," or simply to be liked. Some patients who have been doctoring themselves with homeopathic medicines and supplements, which can change body chemistry, will leave out this vital information. Some who have already diagnosed themselves will recite classic symptoms whether they have these symptoms or not, just to support their own diagnosis. This clouds the issue and further complicates the doctor's assessment. Real honesty is called for here—this is your life at stake.

4. Not providing enough information; being misleading.

A variation of the above, this is where a patient may evaluate the symptoms, prioritize them, and give the doctor only the top several, those bothering him the most. In some cases, particularly with Lyme, it may be the symptoms left out that clinch the diagnosis. This is a good example of where constructing a symptom log/journal will assist the doctor in accurately appraising the situation.

5. Talking too much about irrelevant issues.

One of the signs of disseminated Lyme is that patients tend to suffer from "motor mouth," chatting aimlessly but passionately about their symptoms, their relationships with others, and their treatment at the hands of others. While this can be a red flag for the examining physician, it can also misdirect the doctor's attention if it's done intentionally.

6. Belittling the entire medical profession.

One patient, upon meeting a new doctor, began their interview by telling the doctor what crooks most doctors were, how they charged high prices just to pay for their cars and vacations, and ended with his favorite "joke": "You know what they call a guy who graduates at the bottom of his medical class, don't you? Doctor!" Needless to say, the physician involved was not highly motivated to keep this man as a patient.

Doctors are only human (just ask their spouses!), and treating patients and curing illness is how they make a living. While some do take advantage, most are honestly interested in relieving suffering. They are entitled to charge for their services and will react in a human way when confronted by an obnoxious patient.

7. Patients who take advantage—or just plain take.
People who take objects from the doctor's office, ask to use the doctor's phone for an important call and then conduct business transactions or chat with relatives, or ask for use of the office equipment do nothing to strengthen the doctor-patient partnership.

HOW DOCTORS SABOTAGE THE DOCTOR-PATIENT RELATIONSHIP

1. Doctors frequently don't schedule enough time for patients.
Those doctors who routinely see Lyme disease patients emphasize that the initial visit should take anywhere from one to one and one-half hours. Even on a normal basis, doctors tend to overbook or, giving them the benefit of the doubt, squeeze emergencies into their packed schedules. This leaves sick people sitting in the waiting room for thirty to sixty minutes or more. Then, when the patient finally is seen, the doctor is so frazzled that the patient is rushed through symptoms to "make up" for the tight schedule. This is not a new complaint, but it leads to the next problem.

2. Doctors don't listen.
Surprisingly, many doctors themselves will admit that as a whole, doctors don't listen well. As the patient starts talking, the doctor is already mentally running through disease pathologies to quickly come up with the right answer. Doctors are also often guilty of taking outside calls during an examination, scheduling everything from restaurant reservations to auto repairs, and—

the big problem regarding Lyme—many doctors deny there is even a possibility of Lyme disease and refuse to listen to what their patients have to say about it.

This denial on the part of ill-informed physicians has been responsible for the late diagnosis of Lyme, resulting in the permanent disability of thousands of men, women, and children.

During training, medical students are taught to ask the patient at some point, "What do *you* think the problem is?" Many times, the patient's observations can be helpful in finding the correct diagnosis.

3. Doctors show off to intimidate.

Before Dr. X sees a patient for the first time, the office receptionist hands the patient not only a "new patient information form" but a public relations release on the doctor as well. This lists his accomplishments, speeches, publications, and awards. "By the time the doctor walked in, I felt as though I should stand and applaud," said one, now former, patient, "let alone bother such an important person with my mundane aches and pains."

Although it is important to know that one's doctor is competent, more will be revealed by his willingness to listen to the patient and treat him respectfully than by his using deliberately confusing language, medicalese, and press releases to stun the patient into subservience. An attitude of superiority is a large obstacle to the diagnosis of Lyme—a disease that even the most informed researchers admit is a confusing puzzle. Big egos get in the way of following the clues.

4. Doctors take inadequate medical histories.

"All medical textbooks are written from patient histories," said Debra, a Maryland physician who suffers with Lyme. "I had a medical professor who used to say that all the time, but the fact is, most doctors rush through the history and miss a lot of information that could help them make a good diagnosis. Then the one who pays is the patient."

Since the diagnosis of Lyme is a *clinical one*, the medical history is one of the *most important* diagnostic tools the doctor will have at his disposal. The specifics of what should be included will be discussed later in this chapter.

5. Doctors become defensive when confronted with puzzling symptoms.

Lyme disease is not a snap diagnosis. A doctor cannot take a throat culture, wait fifteen minutes, and pronounce Lyme. It is a painstaking process for both doctor and patient, and there are few patients who can realistically expect a snap answer. Doctors who become defensive when patients suggest Lyme disease reveal more about their own insecurities and inadequacies than anything else. If a doctor reacts in this manner, the whole relationship needs to be reevaluated.

6. Doctors don't believe the patient.

"I told him about the rash and the rest of the symptoms," said Clare. "He told me I must be reading too many newspaper articles."

"I gave my doctor my list of symptoms. She told me that I would be okay when my husband wasn't working the night shift anymore and we had a regular sex life again," said Dina.

"I told the doctor that I keep getting headaches that don't go away, that I had a stiff neck, pain in my knees, and was having trouble reading. And it all started after a field trip to a state park. He told me that being a kid was tough today and that I was just having growing pains," said Mark, a thirteen-year-old Lyme patient.

Unfortunately, these are not isolated incidents. Too many patients report that an early diagnosis (and therefore a cure) was hampered by doctors not believing what they were told. Patients' complaints were dismissed as everything from "growing pains" (kids), to "menopause" (even in women from the late twenties through forty), to stress. It is demeaning to not be believed. More important, if the patient does have Lyme, it is also dangerous.

■ Since the diagnosis for Lyme disease must be a clinical one, both doctors and patients need to polish off their interpersonal skills, throw out all these obstacles to a good working relationship, and strive to form a productive alliance to combat this or any other complicated and puzzling disease.

THE THERAPEUTIC ALLIANCE

Dr. Ken Liegner's office is right in the heart of one of the most beautiful areas of Westchester County, New York—and in one of the country's most hyperendemic areas for Lyme. A member of the medical advisory board for the Lyme Disease Foundation, he has been treating Lyme patients since 1985. His published research has the respect of both academics and clinicians, and his emphasis that Lyme is a clinical diagnosis includes detailed instructions for what he considers the most important diagnostic tool, the patient history, given in the context of a new alliance.

"The therapeutic alliance isn't really a new idea; it stems from psychoanalytic writings stretching way back," he said. "And it should not be unique to Lyme disease. You must have a therapeutic alliance to be successful. A doctor by him- or herself can't do anything; a doctor and patient cooperating can accomplish a lot."

Foremost in developing the alliance on the doctor's side is allowing adequate time for the initial visit and the detailed patient history that must be taken, particularly if there is any question or suspicion of Lyme disease. "Some patients have very long, puzzling histories with symptoms that go over many years and may seem odd. We have to take the time to listen. There is also an art to eliciting a history.

"We are taught in med school to listen to a patient, but a lot of us forget it along the way. We really have to listen carefully to what the patient is saying, not show how smart we are by cutting off their sentence and finishing it. We need to process that information and then ask pointed questions to elicit the kind of information that the patient may not have even realized is important."

This information includes an expanded geographic history of the patient's vocations, vacations, camping and sporting activities, and even daily activities.

One little girl who contracted Lyme was getting progressively sicker. She remained undiagnosed because the physician in charge just couldn't see how, living in a semiurban environment, the child could have been exposed. It wasn't until another physician had her recount a typical day that it was revealed that, in order to catch her school bus, she took a shortcut through two hundred yards of underbrush, stacked wood, and mouse-infested shacks. A subsequent tick collection in that area revealed a high infection rate.

"In order to ask the right questions, a doctor has to have a good understanding of the disease. Because Lyme is so complicated and can present in so many different ways, a doctor has to have a good grasp of the wide range of symptoms that Lyme can produce. The simple, classic symptoms can be recognized by anyone who has bothered to read anything at all on Lyme, but there are so many odd, bizarre, and one-of-a-kind symptoms, a doctor has to at least be aware of the possibilities that exist.

"For this reason, you need a good grasp of medical knowledge generally so you don't go barking up the wrong tree. Just as bad as diagnosing Lyme that isn't there is failing to diagnose a case that is."

Liegner emphasizes that doctors need to return to trusting their own powers of observation—something that makes many of them, who would rather rely on the empirical results of a test, feel uncomfortable. "And a delay in diagnosis can result in long-term, chronic infection," he said. "People need to be made aware of this—both doctors and the general public. Yes, doctors need to be skeptical, especially if they are presented with a patient who has self-diagnosed, but to deny the possibility of Lyme entirely is dangerous and potentially injurious."

■ The medical history, the physical examination, and the relevant tests are all needed to contribute to a diagnosis of Lyme. The most controversial of the three, however, is the testing procedure and its erratic and too frequently unreliable results. In researching Lyme, great emphasis is being placed on discovering reliable tests.

4.
Translating Those Tests into English

The diagnostic problems surrounding Lyme disease are derived primarily from the fact that there have been no tests that could simply and positively detect the *Borrelia burgdorferi* spirochete, thus confirming Lyme and initiating the traditional therapeutic process.

From Tufts University in Massachusettes to Stony Brook in New York to the University of Texas to the NIH-sponsored mecca of scientific research—Rocky Mountain Labs in Hamilton, Montana—specialists from a dozen different fields are pooling their knowledge to pick apart the infectious spirochete, infamous for its ability to transform its appearance chemically, in much the same way a criminal might change clothes and hair color to evade detection and capture.

For this reason, the primary tests for Lyme have measured the body's response to the foreign particles—a measurement of antibodies—rather than picking up the organism itself.

In scientific labs across the country, it has been said that the ideal or "gold standard" test would be to simply be able to grow the *Borrelia burgdorferi* spirochete outside the human body as proof of its presence *in* the body. But, although many bacteria may be able to reproduce every twenty minutes, *B. burgdorferi* has been found to regenerate in a range spanning twelve hours to eighteen days, similar to the rate of the organism that causes TB. In reviewing the damage it inflicts, one can assess just how potent small amounts of this spirochete can be, as well as how difficult it might be to find.

■ Anyone experiencing a difficult-to-diagnose illness becomes conversant in the medical jargon of diagnostic tests, blood counts, and assays (the chemical analyses of substances). Entering the world of Lyme disease is no different. Ranging from the simplest and most commonly used tests to the more complex and more accurate assays currently going through confirmation trials, the tests listed below may assist in determining infection.

THE BASIC TESTS

When infection is present in the human body, the immune system produces complex substances called antibodies to neutralize or destroy the invading organism (the antigen). Each type of antibody, however, recognizes only the type of antigen that provokes its formation. In theory, then, if one were to measure the body's production of Lyme antibodies, it would seem reasonable to assume that Lyme was indeed present.

Three problems arise regarding such a test for Lyme disease, however. The first is that even if you watched a tick that you knew to be infected with *Borrelia burgdorferi* feed on your body for twenty-four hours and then took a blood test, the test would come out negative. This is because it takes the body from three to six weeks or longer to begin to produce the antibodies to fight the infection. During that time, a person can begin to exhibit definite Lyme symptoms, yet will test negative for the disease—despite the fact of sure infection. This would result in a false negative test.

The second problem is that the Lyme spirochete is made up

of thousands of foreign proteins, some of which are similar to the proteins of other bacteria. It is possible that a person with another type of bacterial infection—and who has antibodies to that infection—would test positive for Lyme even if he or she did not have it. This is called cross-reactivity and could result in a false positive test.

Finally, some researchers believe that, particularly in cases where a person was infected months or years prior to the testing, the body's immune system may be so beaten down that only the most highly specialized and sensitive test could detect the antibodies left after the infection has destroyed the original chemical "soldiers."

Further complications arise if the patient has recently taken antibiotics or nonsteroidal anti-inflammatory drugs like ibuprofen, which could inhibit the production of antibodies. New research has shown that the spirochete has the ability to either hide within the cell or change its protein makeup so as to be unrecognizable to the appropriate antibodies. In addition, the reliability of test results is also only as good as the labs and technicians doing the work—various working conditions and mass-produced test kits operate on the sensitivity of the chemicals involved and often produce varied results. More than a few doctors have complained that they have sent portions of the same blood sample to two different labs only to get two different results.

It is obvious, then, why many doctors will either attempt to diagnose Lyme without bothering with antibody tests or will run tests but give little credence to the results.

The most commonly administered tests, if your doctor suspects Lyme could be present, are the IFA, the ELISA, and the Western Blot.

IFA   IFA stands for immunofluorescent assay. This test can be performed with equipment already in place in most laboratories.

It specifically measures total immunoglobulin (Ig), IgM, and IgG (different proteins) antibodies. During various stages of Lyme, the antibody levels will rise. If a patient is presenting arthritic or neurologic symptoms, for example, the IgG or IgM antibody levels could be elevated.

ELISA   This is an enzyme-linked immunosorbent assay, which has been easier to standardize than the IFA and is considered more sensitive. It also tests for IgG and IgM antibodies, indicating their presence through a color change.

Western Blot   This test is often used to confirm borderline-positive serology or in evaluating false positives. It is most useful in revealing the later stages of Lyme disease. It separates the proteins by molecular weight, illustrating them in chartlike bands, some of which are specific for *Borrelia burgdorferi*.

Gundersen Lyme Test   This test was developed by the Gundersen Clinic in La Crosse, Wisconsin, but is not yet readily available throughout the country. It is a very promising test that detects bacteria-killing antibodies found in the blood of Lyme patients. So far, there does not appear to be cross-reactivity. At the time of this writing, the test is undergoing trials in several places.

DETECTION THROUGH DNA

One of the more sensitive tests to be developed is the polymerase chain reaction (PCR), which seeks to identify portions of the DNA (the nucleic acid forming the main component of living cells) from the spirochete itself by using urine, blood, or cerebral spinal fluid samples from the infected patient. Detection of the spirochete's DNA would definitely confirm that a patient has Lyme. The one drawback to PCR, thus far, is that the test itself is so slow (results can take a week) and sensitive that a change of temperature in the lab, the proximity of one specimen to another, and even the level of dust and the technician's handling of the samples can influence the outcome.

Dr. Manfred Bayer is a tall, distinguished-looking scientist who spends his days as director of the Lyme Disease Laboratory of the Fox Chase Institute for Cancer Research in Philadelphia, working through the problems of PCR sensitivity. Bayer, a neurologist specializing in tropical medicine and virology from Hamburg, Germany, is internationally known for his work on bacterial cell surface receptors. Bayer's courtliness doesn't mask the intensity with which he attacks the Lyme disease detection problem. The project is currently being funded by the Prevent Lyme Foundation, the Lyme Disease Coalition of New Jersey, and two private donors.

"There are certain areas of the DNA strand that are very specific to the microorganism from which it comes; other areas are not so specific. We are only interested in the *Borrelia burgdorferi* specific sequences. What one makes is an artificial DNA potion [or probe] that will recognize the specific DNA sequences to that organism [*B. burgdorferi*] taken from the test urine. Normally DNA is double stranded. We need to force it into a single strand [done through a heating process] and at that moment, the complementary artificial piece can find the complementary segment of the bacterial strand."

A continuation of the process involves the adding of an enzyme and several steps of heating and cooling in a reaction chamber; the result is the thousand- to millionfold reproduction of the DNA, which, if from infected fluid, can show spirochetal presence. PCR has allowed scientists to determine that specific portions of the spirochete DNA may affect different portions of the human body.

"There are so many disease possibilities that the physician and scientist must exclude in Lyme disease, and people who are ill may become progressively more devastated," said Bayer. "At what point does PCR become a reliable test? I don't think anyone can answer that yet. We will repeat a dubious positive, but a clinical history has to be considered. PCR alone cannot do the diagnostics right now. The sensitivity of the PCR test is such that all it takes for results to be in question is one unwashed hand grabbing a tube contaminated from an outside source. Sometimes there are lots of these microorganisms out there that can contaminate the sample."

Bayer emphasized that samples for PCR detection must be submitted through a doctor—and only for research purposes at this point, since Fox Chase is not a diagnostic center.

NEW TESTS FROM ROCKY MOUNTAIN LABS

Getting to Rocky Mountain Labs (RML) in Montana is not easy.

A dawn flight from the East Coast takes me to Denver. From Denver, the northward-bound plane descends over an ocean of rugged peaks to land in Bozeman, Montana—well, not actually in Bozeman, a nine-year-old in the seat next to me knowingly explains: "It's just the biggest town closest to the airport." From almost-Bozeman, I fly into Missoula, rent a car, and drive forty minutes to Hamilton.

I try desperately to pay attention to the road instead of the spectacular scenery. As I skid back onto the pavement, I feel like a tiny insect running a maze, surrounded by aloof giants. I pass ranches dotting the sweep up the sides of the mountains, a trio of log homes in progress, and a totem pole carving shop, standing guard over a dozen poles in various stages of emergence.

Finally the town of Hamilton comes into view. Main Street looks like a slightly more developed Cicely, Alaska, from television's popular "Northern Exposure." I ask at the Best Western if the manager knows where Rocky Mountain Labs is. He smiles. "Everyone knows where it is." Just go up the block, turn left, another left, and keep going until you run into it, he says. He doesn't realize he's talking to a person with a retarded sense of direction. I make a dry run so as not to be late for my appointments the next morning.

As I cruise down the tree-lined residential street, the sun dips low enough through the turning leaves to cast an eerie golden glow on the road. I pass from the burnished road to an opening and a cul-de-sac. On my right is a multibuilding complex in red brick, fettered on each end and surrounded on three sides by a high chain-link fence topped with barbed wire. After eleven hours of travel, I have found Rocky Mountain Labs.

It sits with quiet dignity at the end of a street riddled with kids on bikes and pumpkin-faced trash bags filled with leaves. It could be a school, set against the dramatic backdrop of the Rockies. And, in a sense, it is. For what is learned by those who work inside, some of the brightest scientific minds in the country, are the causes and cures of some of the more debilitating and distressing diseases of this century—plague, hepatitis, tuberculosis, AIDS, chlamydia . . . and Lyme disease.

Here is where the ticks, obtained from the canyon visible in the distance, were ground up to make vaccines for Rocky Mountain spotted fever. Here is where a team of sixteen scientists labors full-time, every day, to understand the physiology of the organism so brilliant and virulent that its discoverer, Dr. Willy Burgdorfer, wryly commented, "It's a helluva bug and I'm sorry my name's on it."

Inside the brick building, hunched over a battery of electron microscopes, test tubes, and computer screens, are the scientists like Dr. Richard Marconi, who, through studying RNA ribosomes, has been able to isolate various strains of Lyme disease that will eventually assist in determining treatment, and David Dorward, whose work contributed to the antigen capture test now undergoing trials for reliability and whose fascination with the "dark" side of the organism stems from the recognition that "a healthy human has a very effective immune system. Somehow, this organism can overcome that and then evade being killed."

Then there's Dr. Patti Rosa, for whom spirochetes are practically dinner table conversation, since she is working on studying immune responses and her husband works on Rocky Mountain spotted fever. And there's Dr. William Whitmore, who is very conscious that "people feel science has let them down; they don't see anything happening. But we're all working on pieces of it. Somewhere, a short distance down the road, someone is going to put it all together."

Two tests have recently been produced at RML that look promising for the detection of Lyme disease. One test, currently available, is the recombinant Lyme test (or P-39), developed by Dr. Tom Schwann, and the other, which is in the trial stage, is the antigen capture test, developed by Dr. Claude Garon along with Schwann and Dorward. The first is proving its reliability in testing late-stage Lyme; the second may be a good indicator in the early stages.

The recombinant Lyme test   This test uses DNA from the Lyme spirochete, divided and spliced back together in another bacterium, forcing it to produce a new protein, called P-39, belonging only to *B. burgdorferi*. This protein then causes a strong reaction in cells from Lyme-infected blood.

"We wanted to identify a component of the spirochete that was unique to the Lyme spirochete, that wasn't similar to that in other bacteria," said the youthful Schwann, acting head of the Arthropod-borne Disease Section, Laboratory of Vectors and Pathogens, at RML. "This way, if people had antibodies to this particular component, it would be due to the fact that they had been infected with Lyme, not some other bacteria.

"So far, it's worked beautifully. People who have syphilis don't react, people who have relapsing fever don't react—people who have a whole variety of other bacterial infections don't react to this protein; just those infected with Lyme. I am a strong believer that this test will be great for confirming later-stage Lyme," said Schwann.

Those labs working to conduct continual confirmation trials on the test include the Marshfield Clinic in Wisconsin, the Alfred DuPont Institute in Delaware, and Tufts University.

The antigen capture test   This test detects small blisterlike cells (called *blebs*) given off by the outer membrane of the infectious spirochete. These blebs become free-floating agents and are present in the urine of a patient infected with Lyme.

The assay itself is a two-step procedure employing two different immune system proteins that search out and bind to proteins of the infectious organisms in a manner analogous to a lock and key. The presence of these Lyme proteins is a definite indication of infection.

This assay differs from blood tests now used to diagnose Lyme disease because it detects products of the spirochete rather than the host response to infection.

Dr. Garon, head of both the Structural Pathobiology Section and the Laboratory of Vectors and Pathogens at RML, is intense regarding both the test and the lab's eventual breakdown of the Lyme puzzle.

"When the first word on this test went out, stacks of urine and blood samples arrived every day at the labs. I'd find myself talking on the phone to moms whose children have Lyme disease. It is hard to explain to someone who is going through so much pain that the results of the test aren't going to help that child yet," said Garon. "It looks good, it's working, and now it's going through the necessary trials to make sure that it will be reliable.

"Breakthroughs ride on new techniques and observations. A certain amount of time is built into that, but we are working on it every day. Everyone is involved in a molecular dissection of this bug. We're going to figure out what parts do what so we can come up with something to stop it.

"When polio was a problem, people were looking to build better respirators. One guy, John Enders, was trying to grow monkey cells in a dish. They said he was crazy and wasting his time. The polio vaccine was made possible by growing the virus in monkey cells, modifying the virus, and then injecting people. Then the biggest problem was what to do with warehouses full of iron lungs.

"We will get to the bottom of Lyme disease. Since 1982, RML has published more than one hundred papers on it. The budget for our lab is $1.5 million and more than half goes into Lyme disease research. I think that demonstrates real commitment," said Garon.

"The exciting aspect of the antigen capture test is that if this material is present—whether we are testing urine, blood, or spinal fluid—then infection is present. If the material is gone, then so is the infection. Not only will it be a good diagnostic tool, but we will be able to monitor treatment."

Garon was not sure how long it would be before the test would be widely available, but thought that they might try to bring it out through the veterinary arena since the time element would be shorter.

TESTS FOR DIFFERENTIAL DIAGNOSES

Since your doctor will be attempting to rule out other illnesses in the search for a diagnosis involving Lyme, there are several other tests that are commonly ordered.

Lumbar puncture   Also called a spinal tap, this test is used when there is suspected involvement of the central nervous system. Done under a local anesthetic, it involves withdrawal of fluid with a needle. Doctors are divided over its efficacy·for Lyme, since a negative result does not mean that Lyme isn't present. It is helpful, however, if the infection is being caused by some other infectious agent. The lumbar puncture *is not* done to rule in Lyme, it is done to rule out other diseases.

CAT scan   *CAT* is an abbreviation for computerized axial tomography. This is a painless diagnostic procedure in which hundreds of X rays of a specific area of the body are taken, then fed into a computer, which integrates them to present a very detailed view.

MRI   MRI (magnetic resonance imaging) is a technique based on a computer analysis of the response of atoms of hydrogen, phosphorus, or other elements to a magnetic field. It provides highly detailed visual images of the body and can detect tumors and damaged or diseased tissue.

EEG   This is the electroencephalogram, which, through the measurement of electrical impulses in the brain, rules out abnormal brain activity leading to seizure disorders.

VERS   The VERS, or visual evoked responses, is a more sensitive test for MS.

Blood tests:

> Thyroid profile—to rule out thyroid disease
> ANA—used in collagen diseases, especially lupus
> VDRL-RPR—to rule out syphilis
> CBC—checks for anemia
> B_{12}-folate levels—low levels lead to mental confusion and neurologic defects

The results from any of these tests aside, one aspect of Lyme is finally being recognized as an integral component of this disease. It is, perhaps, the most difficult to measure, the most difficult to accept, and one of the more challenging to treat. This is the psychological aspect of Lyme.

5.
"I'm Not Crazy, I Have Lyme!"

Living in a rural area of Pennsylvania, Lanie loved to spend the time when she wasn't working at the Sylvania plant tending her garden. She thinks that might have been what did her in. First she got severe pain in her joints and pain in her back, then a stiff neck and terrible headaches. Her doctor told the fifty-two-year-old that she had fibrositis, brought on by passing out at the plant and banging her head.

Whatever the cause, Lanie's energy level had been sapped, her production level at work was detrimentally low, and she was experiencing sleep disturbances. She became terribly depressed and cried easily. Her doctor put her on prednisone, muscle relaxers, and sleeping pills, but her body continued to fall apart. Pressing for a reevaluation, she was told she had fibromyalgia and depression and that she'd have to live with them.

"My husband, who was having similar symptoms, was going to retire to take care of me," she said. "I kept having more symptoms and thought I was going to lose my mind. I had stomach pain, my arms were getting weak. The doctor didn't believe me. I had a wonderful life and it was falling apart." Then she saw an article in *Outdoor Life* magazine on Lyme disease and her symptoms began to fall into place. She sought out a Lyme support group, even though it met more than a hundred miles from her home, and listened to an epidemiologist give a presentation that opened her eyes further. Most of those Lyme patients had to travel out of state for knowledgeable treatment.

She went to see her local doctor again and he gave her ulcer medication. "I asked for a Lyme test and he told me he didn't want to even discuss it. He said I was being ridiculous."

Lanie returned home, feeling demoralized. She took the medicine for her stomach and reacted with Bell's palsy. She called another doctor, who recommended a spinal tap. When she asked if she could have a Lyme test, he said, "If you think you know more than I do, go find yourself another doctor."

"Then I had no doctor, and no one who could tell me about Lyme. I was so nervous by that time, I was dealing with such pain and pressure in my head, that I just snapped one afternoon. I started to cry hysterically on the back porch—everything just seemed to come crashing down on me and I had to let it out. Well, the neighbors heard me wailing and called the police. When the police came, they pushed me down on the ground and put me in a straitjacket. I kept yelling at them, 'I'm not crazy! I have Lyme disease, I have Lyme disease!' but they wouldn't listen. They drove me to the county hospital and put me on the psycho ward.

"They got ahold of my husband, but it didn't do any good. I had to stay there for five days, by law, before they could let me out. They wanted to do an evaluation. They gave me Compazine and Elavil, and I had an allergic reaction to the Compazine— my tongue swelled and I could hardly breathe. The psychiatrist came in and scolded me that if I didn't stop complaining, he was going to confine me to the state mental hospital.

"While I was there, a medical student who was working there came to see me. He said he had the same kind of symptoms I had and we compared notes. Finally, on the fifth day, my husband came with a lawyer who confronted the doctors with all kinds of supportive information on Lyme and they let me out.

"I finally got to a doctor—had to go to Indiana—and began treatment. You really are treated as if you are crazy, and you begin to doubt your own sanity. Some days it was really hard to hang on."

■ Not all tales are as dramatic as Lanie's, but talk to a thousand Lyme patients and you will get a thousand variations of the same story: people who are normally easygoing become moody and belligerent; those who are outgoing become lethargic; mood swings cause the breakup of marriages and career relationships; the inability to concentrate results in job losses, plunging grades in school, and accidents; short-term memory loss affects habits and speech; and everywhere there is depression, a loss of self-esteem, and suicidal thoughts from people who have never had a history of such things.

Like that other infamous spirochetal illness, syphilis, Lyme disease has a definitive array of psychological symptoms as well as physical ones. Depending upon the lag time between the tick bite and treatment, these symptoms can be either mild or severe.

The symptoms, coupled with all the other reasons for misdiagnosis and late diagnosis, often prompt doctors to tell Lyme patients, "Look, there's nothing wrong with you physically— it's all in your head. Go see a psychiatrist." This scenario has been replayed with such frequency that it has become a standing joke among Lyme patients: they say that if your doctor finally tells you to go see a shrink, that's the confirmation that you have Lyme disease! And as one psychiatrist wryly commented, "We are at the end of a long line of doctors. When nobody else can figure out what's wrong with a patient, they send him to us."

Far from being humorous, however, the mind-body connection is one of the more difficult aspects with which to deal, both when seeking a proper diagnosis and when just attempting to cope on a daily basis. The Lyme infection apparently wreaks havoc with those neurons affecting the personality and emotional balance.

Contrary to a prevailing belief, those who are felled by Lyme are not hypochondriacs looking for attention. In fact, there is a lot of denial that goes on—first over physical symptoms, then when the possibility of Lyme disease arises, and finally when psychological symptoms appear. This is not only a threatening aspect of the illness itself, but if the patient has had to fight for a diagnosis and treatment, the vicious cycle of doubt, self-doubt, and alienation and depression figures largely into the struggle for regaining health.

This is difficult enough for an adult who has a track record of wellness and a strong identity to fall back on, but when Lyme attacks children and teens the psychological presentations are intermingled with a number of other developmental issues. So while all of the following symptoms apply to young people as well, I will deal with the specific psychological effects and symptoms of Lyme on children and teens in chapters 7 and 8.

ZEROING IN ON THE PSYCHOLOGICAL ASPECTS

"When I asked for a Lyme test, the doctor asked me if I was afraid that my husband was going to leave me," said thirty-two-year-old Linda, who had been suffering with fatigue, joint pain, headaches, and swollen glands. "She said my symptoms were psychosomatic and would go away when our sex life picked up.

"I remember being on a school trip with my daughter on the bus and suddenly I felt as though I was in a fog and everyone else was far away. I could hear the noise and it was irritating, but I couldn't connect. I thought, 'My God, I *am* going crazy.' When a doctor tells you, 'It's all in your head,' you try to justify all your symptoms.

"It took two years and five doctors to figure out I had Lyme disease. It put a strain on my marriage, on my family relationships, and there were times that I was so depressed that

I wondered if I'd finish out my days in the cuckoo ward. I've lost friends, self-esteem, and two years of my life, and I'm just hoping that someday soon I'll get back to normal. I ran into that first doctor recently. When I told her that I was being successfully treated for Lyme, she told me that I was crazy. That I didn't have Lyme disease and never did."

■ Fortunately for Lyme patients like Linda, doctors are beginning to realize that Lyme disease does cause certain psychological changes with which one must be prepared to deal. A good portion of the credit for bringing this to the attention of the medical community goes to Dr. Brian Fallon, an NIH fellow with the New York State Psychiatric Institute at Columbia University in New York City, who has made the psychiatric aspects of Lyme disease a passionate area of study.

It began with a flood of referrals from doctors who couldn't figure out what was wrong with their patients and thus concluded "it must be in their heads." He has now presented papers at medical conferences both in the United States and in Europe, and has, together with Drs. Burrascano, Liegner, and Jennifer Nields, initiated surveys and studies that are serving as the yardstick for evaluating Lyme patients psychologically.

Based on treatment experience and the results of the nationally distributed survey, the psychological symptoms of Lyme include:

- Major depression
- Extreme fatigue
- Emotional instability (crying easily)
- Increased irritability and mood swings
- Sensitivity to light
- Sleep disturbances (insomnia; too much sleep)
- Memory problems

- Getting lost in familiar places
- Dyslexia-type reversals
- Significant loss of libido
- Night terrors
- Panic attacks
- Ferocious nightmares
- Suicidal thoughts
- Mental fog
- Disorientation
- Feelings of rage
- Violent thoughts
- Abnormalities of taste
- Abnormalities of smell
- Heightened sensitivity to vibrations and noise
- Depersonalization
- Spatial problems
- Appetite changes (bulimia, anorexia)

Secondary psychological problems arising from Lyme include feelings of inadequacy, low self-esteem, bitterness, guilt, and alienation, as well as doubting one's sanity ("I feel as though I'm losing my mind" is a commonly heard phrase).

"The experience of Lyme is such that a patient will have unusual symptoms to the point of being disbelieved by doctors and family and finally disbelieving him- or herself," said Fallon. "This disease follows a waxing and waning course. You can't predict how you're going to feel the next day, next month, or next year. Family, friends, and schools say, 'Why are you okay one day and not the next?' Add to this that many patients have negative blood tests so there may be uncertainty of a Lyme diagnosis, and then you also have fear—fear of losing one's job, fear of losing health, and fear of losing the support of family and friends who may be supportive during the first month of the illness, but when this goes on and on, friends and family may get pretty tired of it.

"Lyme patients also feel a loss of control, not only of their bodies and feelings, but also the ability to anticipate and predict the future. Then they deal with shame, guilt, and finally anger directed at doctors and family members."

"Often psychiatrists are being asked to see these patients before a diagnosis of Lyme disease is made," said Fallon. "Incorrectly labeling these patients as having functional depression or hypochondriasis or a somatization disorder may result in delayed antibiotic treatment. Such a delay can lead to further dissemination of infection, severe disability, and possible chronic neurological damage.

"Because of the rapid increase of Lyme disease in the country, it's important for mental health professionals as well as other health professionals to be aware of these psychological manifestations. Oftentimes, if you don't have the advantage of the tick bite and rash, these patients aren't picked up as having Lyme disease until too late."

Although the psychological manifestations of the disease are dismissed by some as "Lyme anxiety," that term cannot begin to cover the varied and intense personality changes that accompany Lyme, particularly in people who have no history of those types of changes. *The most common presentation is a feeling of depression.* And although some may simply experience uncomfortable feelings of doom, others experience a more sustained version, even to the point of gross debilitation.

LYME AND DEPRESSION

In an article for *Emergency Medicine*, Dr. Edwin H. Cassem, chief of psychiatry at Massachusetts General Hospital in Boston and professor of psychiatry at Harvard Medical School, wrote that classic depression has eight specific criteria, which he reduced to a mnemonic: Sig E. Caps (a doctor's prescription for energy capsules). This stands for *sleep, interest, guilt, energy, concentration, appetite, psychomotor,* and *suicidal ideas.* If a patient displays symptoms in four of the eight areas, he or she meets the criteria for major depression.

According to Fallon's study, which was done only on seropositive patients, 85 percent experienced sleep disturbances; 94 percent experienced extreme fatigue; 84 percent suffered from irritability and agitation; 24 percent had worked through suicidal plans, while many more admitted to suicidal thoughts; and 83 percent had difficulty with concentration and memory. Although specific questions regarding interests were not posed, most patients reported a significant loss of libido and interest in other aspects of their lives. Most also commented on the guilt they felt for the length of time they were ill; for the physical, emotional, and financial toll their illness was taking on their families; and for not being able to "will" themselves well. And just as with the physical presentations of Lyme, the psychological disturbances affect a patient's whole family.

Tom found his diagnosis on a milk carton. The thirty-eight-year-old was a self-employed furniture maker who loved to camp and study ecology with an artisan's eye. It could have been during one of his forays into the countryside or even while coaching his Little League team that Tom was bitten by the tick. As both his body and personality deteriorated (he was so dizzy, he felt "high" all the time), he made the rounds of doctors who threw tranquilizers at him to help him cope with "stress." By this time, the pressure in his head was so bad that he would curl up on the floor in a fetal position and cry. He couldn't bear noise and would lash out at those closest to him for the simplest comments or questions.

When he saw Lyme disease information on a milk carton

one morning, a light went on. Tom finally found a knowledge-able doctor and began treatment, but ask any member of his family what it is like to have someone with Lyme in the house and there is a tussle over who'll answer first. "I hate it," the thirteen-year-old says angrily. "It's the pits," admits Tom's wife. "I don't even want to think about it," agrees the nine-year-old.

"This kind of thing, it affects families for life," says Tom's wife, Di. "The kids never know what kind of mood he's going to be in, so everyone walks on eggshells. The youngest one now hits himself in the head when he gets frustrated because he saw his father do that so often. I got to the point that I was crying all the time.

"One of the hardest things to deal with is that he doesn't *look* sick. Sick people are supposed to look sick, and everyone has sympathy for them. With Lyme, you can look pretty normal even though your body and mind seem to be falling apart on the inside, and people think you're a hypochondriac, making up symptoms."

Not being believed because one doesn't "look sick" adds to the Lyme patient's frustrations and self-doubts, but the lack of control over one's body—and mind—adds to overall depression.

Scott also does not look sick. In fact, if one were to look around a room full of people, this muscular man with blond hair, clear skin, and an engaging smile would be last on your list of sickly types. But for the last two years he has waged a battle with Lyme that has taken a toll both physically and emotionally.

"I was driving down a street in my neighborhood, where I've lived all my life," said the twenty-seven-year-old, who owns and operates his own landscaping business. "And suddenly, I was lost! I didn't recognize a thing. That is so scary! I mean, I lived on that street for years, and in an instant, I couldn't figure out where I was. I know of another guy with Lyme who put his hand on the doorknob and suddenly he couldn't remember how to turn the key to open the door. When these kinds of things happen, you really have to fight to remain stable. You go from being an active, competent person to being afraid to go out and even be with people because you don't know if you're going to forget words when you open your mouth."

This uncertainty and lack of control have forced many adult Lyme patients back into a dependent position, whether living at their parents' home again or simply having to depend on others in the household to do the simplest personal tasks. This contributes to feelings of guilt, worthlessness, and resentment, which can spill over onto the very people who are helping. Adding to the difficulty with relationships is the loss of libido that many people experience.

LOSS OF LIBIDO

"I feel as though I've been castrated," said Kelly, a very attractive thirty-something mother of three who has suffered with Lyme for the last four years. "I know that sounds funny coming from a woman, but that tick took more away from me than just my good health and sanity. I can't tell you the problems it has caused between my husband and me. He kept thinking I was pushing him away, and I was trying to convince him that I was in *pain* and sex was the last thing on my mind.

"When he gave me an ultimatum, I finally told him if it was that important to him, go get 'it' someplace else and leave me alone. I don't think he did, but what's more shocking to me is that I actually said those words to him. I mean, I love my husband—he has always been my best friend and support. Sometimes I think I'm really going crazy and then I get depressed."

Patients report that not only do they tend to lose interest in sex, but that their sex lives also suffer as a result of the mood swings and verbal backlash that strain a close relationship. "A lot of what goes on under the sheets starts with the interaction and feelings that are generated when two people aren't anywhere near the bedroom," said one man. "You have someone who is going off the wall emotionally, being verbally abusive one minute and then critical or ultrasensitive the next—well, even if he *is* interested in sex, chances are his partner won't be because of hurt feelings and hostility. And that causes all kinds of problems as well."

As if all of this isn't enough to contend with, Lyme can both trigger and/or mask other psychological syndromes.

WHAT ELSE CAN POSSIBLY GO WRONG?

Harry had been fighting Lyme for more than two years. Diagnosed late and displaying many neurological symptoms, he was under a doctor's care when his wife noticed that he was becoming obsessive about bugs. He'd look everywhere for them when he entered a room. He wouldn't sit in a chair until he had inspected it with a magnifying glass for ticks, and he meticulously checked all the food served to him, both at home and in restaurants, to the point of continuing to examine his food when everyone else was done.

Harry was diagnosed as having obsessive-compulsive disorder (OCD), but the doctor admits that he can't tell whether it was caused by the Lyme or whether Harry just falls into the 2 to 3 percent of the population that suffers from this disorder naturally.

Surely, it does not seem unreasonable that a person, after suffering with Lyme, becomes a little paranoid about checking for ticks. But OCD also precipitates weird thoughts that make no sense, said Dr. Fallon. These thoughts can be about anything from germs to sexually related situations to aggression.

Apart from true clinical depression, another psychological factor that is being mentioned in relation to Lyme disease is the "rage response." This is displayed primarily by males from adolescence to adulthood, and stories abound of fists being put through walls, heavy objects being lifted and thrown, and formerly docile people becoming enraged disproportionately to the given situation. Although sheer frustration over the other manifestations of the illness, the lack of diagnosis, and perhaps lack of immediate response to treatment would seem enough to provoke extreme anger, psychiatrists say that the cause could also be a temporal lobe seizure. This, like OCD, requires close scrutiny and evaluation by a psychiatrist.

Finally, at some point, most chronic Lyme patients get angry. This anger may be directed at the medical profession for not recognizing and treating the problem and thus preventing a chronic condition; it could be directed at those closest to them, for not being able to understand their pain or simply for being well; and it could be directed at themselves, for having the disease.

Scott has found an outlet for his anger—he brainstorms ideas for either curing Lyme or trying to work the bugs out of the current system of medical management.

"You have to take the anger and find a way to make it work," he said with thoughtful determination. "For example, if it's so much trouble for doctors to fill out a report form on Lyme disease, why can't they just Xerox the insurance form they fill out with the recommended tests and diagnosis and submit that? That would give the CDC and government agencies an accurate record of who is being treated. This is the kind of thing I try to think about—coming up with solutions and contacting the people in charge. This disease has changed me. I used to be a high-stress person, rushing through my day. Now I appreciate little things; the hours when I feel good, and taking the time to listen to people and the world around me.

"When they finally find a cure for Lyme disease, I'm going to be so happy. And I'll be glad at that point that I had this experience, because I'll be stronger mentally and emotionally than other people. All of us will who have been through this. We've had to be to survive."

"A certain amount of anger is not all bad," said Fallon. "Everyone deals with it in a different way. Some intellectualize it, and some displace it. But everyone needs a support and information network where they can work this out of their systems. The bottom line is that you have to be your own advocate and search for your health—your physical and mental health."

COPING AND SURVIVING

Dr. Richard Goldman, a veterinarian who has struggled back from the brink of blindness and despondency with Lyme, says, "Patience is not a virtue—it's a survival tool if you have Lyme disease!" Although it is difficult to infuse someone else with patience, Kathy Cavert, an R.N. with Lyme, who publishes *LymeAid* out of Independence, Missouri, has used her extensive psychological training and experience to offer some practical coping skills to Lyme patients. Ranging from the physical to the spiritual, Kathy's tips can be condensed to the mnemonic FACE PEG:

Flexibility   Also called "rolling with the punches." Lyme patients must recognize that rigid rules of life need to be set aside if they are going to cope successfully and win out over this relapsing and remitting disease.

Awareness   Not only of one's mortality but of the choice one has to make whether to rely on external sources for satisfaction or on internal sources. "This is referred to as the external locus of control versus the internal," says Kathy. "The internal control is very powerful as we depend upon our own strengths and resources to stay afloat. We can be sorely disappointed if we let our external environment control our feelings."

Counseling Not only is counseling essential for those who were dealing with physical and emotional problems prior to contracting Lyme, it is also an emotional handrail for those who are feeling their way through this confusing and frustrating illness. The need for reassurance is great and short-term counseling has been proven to be of great benefit in marshaling a person's internal resources.

Education The disease becomes much less mysterious when one makes an effort to understand the clinical symptoms and signs. In addition, a Lyme patient must be a vigilant medical consumer in order to obtain the best care available and not be led astray by agencies or doctors who are unaware.

Pacing This is a way of saving energy, preventing overfatigue and possible injury, and being able to live as normal a life as possible. Lyme patients may have to realize that while they have an active case of Lyme they may not be able to work as many hours, stay out as late, or even accomplish the same number of tasks in a day as they did prior to Lyme.

Exercise Increasingly, knowledgeable doctors like Joe Burrascano are recommending regular regimens of aerobic exercise for their Lyme patients, even if that means following a brief exercise period with a nap. Not only does exercise raise the body temperature and suppress some of the more bothersome symptoms, it is good therapy for the mind as well. In fact, even those Lyme patients who have difficulty with the arthritic component of the disease report that strenuous physical exercise makes them feel better.

Giving It is easy to fall into the pit of self-absorption. After all, with the plethora of aches and pains and life-style changes Lyme may inflict, the tendency for preoccupation with one's own health looms large. To get on with life and put those pains in perspective, get out of the house, call a friend, volunteer some time answering the telephone at a literacy program—do something to remind yourself that a lot of other people out there need help too.

■ Finally, have faith—in the fact that you are not alone in this illness, in the fact that there are many people who are waging the battle against Lyme, and in yourself. You are not going crazy; you just have Lyme disease.

Having faith is admittedly more difficult for a patient when a doctor misses the diagnosis. It is equally difficult for a doctor when the government or a public health department refuses to validate his or her diagnosis. Both doctors and patients are recognizing that despite the growing recognition of Lyme disease, it is still a political football.

6.

The Politics of Diagnosing Lyme Disease

The Department of Health for the state of Florida officially denies the presence of Lyme disease in this tourist-oriented playground. Yet a Gainesville veterinarian, who came close to losing his eyesight and his practice because of Lyme, counsels hundreds of callers per month who exhibit the classic symptoms and are desperately and fruitlessly searching for a doctor who can and will help them. A good number of these calls come from out-of-state victims who contracted Lyme while on a Florida vacation, as well as from those who are residents of the state. This volume is at least duplicated in South Florida, where a neuroophthalmologist at the University of Miami's Bascom-Palmer Institute has documented several hundred cases of Lyme.

■ The Centers for Disease Control specifically warns that its case description for Lyme disease is strictly for epidemiological tracking and is not to be used as a guideline for diagnosis. Yet in a letter to Ken Fordyce, head of New Jersey's Governor's Council on Lyme Disease, the medical director for Blue Cross and Blue Shield, responding to a request for justification of terminating clients' coverage for Lyme disease treatment, said: "To assess medical evidence, we begin by trying to establish the case definition as defined by the Centers for Disease Control."

■ The Missouri Department of Health sent this directive to one of the more active physician-researchers in Lyme today, Dr. Edwin Masters: "It would be wise to call this Lyme-like illness rather than Lyme disease." Masters, frustrated after five years of meticulously documenting hundreds of cases, says, "Lyme disease is a clinical diagnosis until you make it. Then it's not a clinical diagnosis—it's a political diagnosis!"

■ To many clinicians and patients across the country, the politics of diagnosing Lyme disease is similar to the politics surrounding the acknowledgment of another monumental hazard, albeit fictional.

When the great white shark of *Jaws* fame relentlessly feasted on unsuspecting bathers off the shores of the fictional town of Amity, the reactions ranged from the hysteria of those who saw sharks in every ripple of the water's surface to denial by the town fathers that anything unusual had occurred. The official thinking went: If we don't acknowledge the shark, then tourists won't stay away and we won't have a problem. Today, we are suffering from that same "Amity mentality," but the shark is Lyme disease, and the consequences are not fictional.

From California to Tennessee and Texas to the Carolinas, Lyme disease sufferers have been forced to travel hundreds of miles—often out of state—on a regular basis for treatment because of medical ignorance and hostility or the governmental fear that acknowledging Lyme disease would be injurious to the economic vitality of an area. The prevailing "Amity-speak" at work here is: If we don't acknowledge Lyme disease, then doctors won't look for it, so there will be no Lyme disease.

But, of course, Lyme disease does exist, and this roadblock to immediate and efficient health care has inspired a groundswell of medical consumer activism paralleling the early AIDS demonstrations, networks, confrontations, and legislation.

Like AIDS, chronic Lyme disease at present has no cure, and treatment can be expensive and sometimes controversial. In addition, its comparison to another relapsing and remitting spirochetal illness—syphilis—inspires a negative attitude among medical representatives because the disease does not respond to the officially endorsed treatment. And city fathers view it negatively because this is an infection borne not by an individual's behavior but by environmental agents, and *nobody* wants to be "blamed" for a hazard. The irony is that, the way Lyme disease is spreading, the question of where one acquired it will be moot. The focus needs to be on who is going to provide the most efficient diagnosis and treatment before growing numbers of debilitated citizens are denied the chance to live normal lives.

REPORTING = LOOKING = REPORTING

Like most nine-year-olds, Mandy loved Halloween. She especially looked forward to her trip to the local pumpkin farm to pick out just the right one for her family's jack-o'-lantern.

After a trip to the pumpkin farm in 1988, however, she developed a rash. Her mother informed doctors about the rash but was told not to worry, as rashes are a common and minor affliction in rural New Jersey. Then came a series of increasing complaints of blistering headaches, painful joints, and other symptoms from the young girl, who was normally outgoing, friendly, and active. After six months of increasing debilitation, Mandy slipped into a coma. Her mother begged the doctors to administer a Lyme test. They refused, brushing her off with denials of Lyme disease's existence. Mandy's mother didn't give up.

Finally, when the little girl came out of the coma, the Lyme test was given. Mandy was positive, but antibiotics prolonged her life for only eighteen months. Mandy died because of swelling of her brain due to Lyme disease. Hers was a death that could have been avoided.

"Somebody should have said, 'Let's try antibiotics at this time,' but they were too busy telling us it wasn't Lyme," said Mandy's mother in an article for the *Trentonian* newspaper.

Some may argue that not much was known about Lyme disease back in 1988, that what happened to Mandy would not happen today. Unfortunately, nothing is further from the truth. Despite the fact that the CDC has been tracking Lyme for ten years and that there has been a recent "discovery" of Lyme by both public health officials and the media, this disease is in its infancy in terms of our understanding of how it operates, how to get rid of it, and how to educate both the public and those who have the power to help eradicate it.

"Our job is to protect the public health—disease prevention and control," said Dr. David Dennis, director of the CDC Lyme Disease Project, in operation since 1989. "The problem is, with Lyme disease we don't have a proper tool at the present time to say 'Yes, this is definitely Lyme' or 'No, this definitely is not Lyme.' "

To come up with the current case definition of Lyme, the CDC convened a group of experts from various scientific disciplines to formulate a description that could be used as a standard across the United States for tracking the growth of the disease. This description is admittedly bare-bones, according to Dennis, and leaves out many of the variations that Lyme disease includes. For this reason, the CDC warns doctors and insurance companies repeatedly not to use its case definition for diagnostic and evaluation purposes. In fact, due to the explosion of Lyme disease cases across the country, sometime in 1993 the CDC will be changing its surveillance criteria to possibly include additional descriptors.

The Lyme disease national surveillance case definition, until that change, is as follows:

1. A person with erythema migrans (rash); or
2. A person with at least one late manifestation and laboratory confirmation of infection.

As was previously stated, however, not everyone gets or remembers a rash, and the current serologic tests have been unreliable. Using only these two criteria to describe Lyme is like having every town report how many apples it has, with the definition of apples being only that they are solid red in color and have a diameter of three inches.

"The diagnosis of Lyme disease has to be a clinical diagnosis," emphasized Dennis, "meaning that doctors should use the tests as just another tool when considering a diagnosis of Lyme. For tracking purposes, we have to make sure each case is exactly alike, even if that represents only a small number. But we encourage doctors to report *all* cases of Lyme disease to their health departments. Many states have a two-drawer system; one drawer for the ones that fit our strict criteria, and one for all the others. But none of that works if we can't get doctors to report it."

The Lyme disease case report is a simple, one-page, twenty-five-question form. Why don't doctors report? Like the disease, the answers can be complicated.

There are always those doctors who retort: "It takes too much time" and "I hate doing paperwork."

There are a good number who are frustrated at attempting to report cases of Lyme disease; if a case does not match the CDC criteria, it is refused by the health department. Runarounds at various health departments, according to doctors surveyed, also include being put on "hold" when mentioning Lyme disease, being told that nobody there is assigned to handle Lyme, and

being referred from clerk to clerk until the telephone is discon-
nected.

There are also doctors, such as those in the hyperendemic
section of southern New Jersey, who are threatened by insurance
companies for overreporting Lyme disease. As was explained in
the *Asbury Park Press*, doctors who reported large numbers of
Lyme disease cases would be in danger of having their medical
licenses lifted pending an investigation. This type of scare tactic
levied by the larger insurance carriers tends to motivate doctors
to refer suspected Lyme cases to other physicians rather than
diagnose, report, and treat.

All of the above factors lead many physicians to stop short
of reporting Lyme, concluding: "It really doesn't matter anyway."

They are wrong. Reporting Lyme disease *does* matter.

Underreporting of a disease leads to more "Amity-speak":
if we underreport, then there is no problem, so there is no need
for funding to find a cure for a problem that does not exist.
Witness Health Secretary Joseph Califano's early press conference during President Bill Clinton's transition into the White
House. Califano emphasized that the main focus in government
funding will be on AIDS, substance abuse, and tuberculosis. The
spread of Lyme disease, which, in its late stages, resists treatment,
needs to be addressed as well.

Underreporting matters to patients like Lillith, in South
Carolina, who began having to travel to New Jersey for Lyme
treatment when her own doctor, bowing to pressure from his
partners, told her that after two months of treatment she "should
be cured of a disease that doesn't really affect the Carolinas
anyway."

It matters to patients like fourteen-year-old Corey, who
went from being an achiever both on and off the basketball court
to being unable to walk across a room without trembling and

tripping, and whose New York doctor refused to see him in 1990 when his mother called to report the rash and other symptoms, stating, "This Lyme disease is just a bunch of hysteria. Don't worry about it." Corey now has permanent damage to his brain and his heart as a result of a late diagnosis.

Reporting the disease matters to health departments, both in endemic states like Connecticut, Rhode Island, Wisconsin, and New Jersey and in those other states where Lyme is spreading like wildfire and is competing for public health dollars with AIDS, tuberculosis, and other infectious diseases. Reporting also serves to remind health departments that ticks cannot read state border signs, and that they continually cross into areas where they "are not supposed to be."

And it matters to those doctors who are running themselves into the ground treating Lyme patients in the face of suspicion and criticism from academic circles and many peers who have fallen victim to the prevailing "Amity-speak."

TRACKING A LYME-LIKE ILLNESS

Mark Twain would have been comfortable in Cape Girardeau, Missouri. Perched on the banks of the Mississippi River, the town provides its farmers and friendly residents a view clear across to Illinois and, on an inspired day, maybe even to Kentucky. These are hardworking people who don't stop to complain about little aches and pains, and certainly not rashes, as they toil during the week to put food on the table and enjoy the small-town life with their families on the weekends.

Dr. Edwin Masters, of Cape Girardeau, describes himself as a "simple country doc," but his quick grin and folksy homilies can't hide his acuity and concern when discussing the nearly one thousand cases of the disease he has diagnosed but cannot get his state to recognize.

"I'm a tree farmer by avocation, so when the state medical society was holding a conference, they asked me to prepare a talk on Lyme disease. Hell, I didn't know anything about Lyme, and I didn't believe it existed in these parts, but I operate on Masters's Maxim—that is, anything that's worth doing is worth overdoing. I collected hundreds of articles, prepared slides, studied, and presented my findings at the meeting."

That was the beginning of a five-year crusade, but the major obstacle was the fact that the *Ixodes dammini* tick, the primary Lyme vector, was not common in Missouri.

"Suddenly, certain illnesses and symptoms I had been seeing began falling into place," said Masters. "I had patients who came in with these look-alike bull's-eye rashes, and look-alike spirochetes, and look-alike symptoms, so I made look-alike diagnoses. But when I questioned them about tick bites, the ticks they described were often the size of a watermelon seed with a white spot in the middle. I was the most skeptical of all, but these were farmers, school kids, old ladies, laborers—people who wouldn't know an *Amblyomma americanum* [Lone Star tick] from Godzilla, yet they were all describing the same thing! I thought, 'How can this be?'"

Continuing to operate on Masters's Maxim, he discovered that Missouri is directly in the path of one of the greatest flyways in the country, where millions of migratory birds land in their treks from north to south and back again. Not only were the birds pausing to refresh themselves in Missouri, they apparently were also depositing infected ticks along their migratory path.

Masters meticulously photographs and cultures his patients' rashes, and he also keeps both blood and urine samples on all of his suspected Lyme disease cases. According to the state and CDC, he can attribute the cases only to a Lyme-like illness, despite the documentation of classic symptoms and classic responses to antibiotics. The stumbling block, according to Dr. Dennis, who heads the CDC Lyme Disease Project, is that the

CDC has not been able to grow *Borrelia burgdorferi* in a specifically employed medium. Masters maintains that the different strains of Lyme that researchers have been discovering and the fact that the Missouri Lyme is apparently contracted from a different type of tick could be factors here.

"We have a lot of patients falling through the cracks, and those cracks extend from Indiana to Nebraska and Iowa to Texas," said Masters. "This 'Lyme-like' illness needs a name. I'm a country doc in a small town and I have to see these suffering patients. I can't give them two weeks of whatever treatment, then close my eyes and say, 'You are cured. Go away. Go see a psychiatrist and don't bug me.' I have to live with these people, and they come back! I have to call it like I see it. These people are sick, and they deserve to be treated."

The Missouri story is not dissimilar to the situations found in states from Tennessee and Kentucky to Alabama and Florida and the Virginias. Again, patients were turning up in droves with classic Lyme symptoms but being turned away by doctors who had been told the disease did not exist outside of the Northeast. This contradiction came to the attention of Southeast Outdoor Press Association (SEOPA) members, whose professional and recreational lives revolve around the enjoyment of outdoor sports, including hunting, fishing, camping, gaming, and hiking. Not only were these men and women struggling to bring the tick-borne disease to the public's and the medical profession's attention—by filing numerous stories on this illness contracted by those who worked out-of-doors, such as farmers, utility workers, and parks and landscape professionals—many of the press members themselves began falling victim to Lyme disease. The result was the creation of a specially organized effort.

"Last year in South Carolina, SEOPA decided to take a more activist part in educating people about Lyme disease," said Norris Blackburn, a resident of Morristown, Tennessee, and a former SEOPA president. "We need to educate physicians as well as the public because doctors are seeing more of this than ever before, but aren't recognizing it until the patient slips into the late or chronic stage and is affected for life. We are going to be staging major efforts to bring the true facts about Lyme disease to the attention of the medical profession and urge that something be done."

Part of that "something" revolves around documentation of vectors and levels of infection in a specific geographic area, to gain the CDC's acknowledgment of a Lyme disease problem in that area. This type of painstaking work began as an intriguing intellectual exercise for Dr. James Oliver, professor of biology and director of arthropodology and parisitology for Georgia Southern University. Like Masters, however, Dr. Oliver is now a passionate laborer in the Lyme disease arena, after witnessing the unrelenting pain and suffering that was going unheeded.

"The CDC is conservative, and rightly so, because they don't want a panic developing, but those people with increasing symptoms are becoming distraught. This is such a diffuse issue: we have the awareness versus unawareness and the need for research-type studies. The problem with getting study participants is, when a patient is ill and goes to his doctor, the doctor can say, 'Well, I think this is Lyme disease and I can prescribe an antibiotic to start you getting well, or we can enroll you in this study and over the course of the next twelve to twenty-four weeks your symptoms will be studied and some of you will be given antibiotics.' Which way do you think the patient is going to go?"

Another problem in Georgia, as in Missouri, is that the Lyme-carrying *Ixodes* tick was rare, despite the increasing number of Lyme cases. So Oliver meticulously documented, by DNA-sequencing probes, that the infected black-legged tick was the same as the *Ixodes*, isolating it in four large geographic locations from the northern part of Georgia to Cape Canaveral in Florida.

His research was presented at the Fifth International Conference on Lyme Disease, sponsored by the NIH, thus opening the door for official recognition of the disease. This is still slow in coming.

"I think we have to go with the caveat that with all we still don't know about Lyme disease, maybe all the last *i*'s aren't dotted when people are suffering but we still need to treat them. Sure, we may actually be treating a few people who don't have it, but is that worse than missing the many who are suffering and sliding into chronic illness? I don't think so."

This is a sentiment expressed by many who are in the midst of the Lyme battle, but it is not one eagerly embraced by the medical profession overall. At least, not among the more vocal conservatives.

THE POLITICS OF THE MEDICAL PROFESSION

During the mid-1970s, hospitals across the country were seeing thousands of patients complaining of extreme stomach pain, many of them in such pain that they couldn't function. Surgery was commonplace. Then, a drug named Tagamet was discovered. Upon being administered, this drug relieved the stomach distress, and surgery rates dropped. It was a dramatic discovery, and soon Tagamet became the number one prescribed drug in the country, with patients actively seeking it out.

However, doctors were told that they could prescribe Tagamet for only two weeks, or they would be considered "cowboys" or wild doctors. The patients, sliding back into pain and dysfunction, continued seeking out new doctors to prescribe the drug so they could continue with their lives. Fifteen years later, medical science decided that the patients were right all along, and now doctors routinely prescribe Tagamet for prolonged periods of time.

This particular case illustrates the slowness with which the medical profession, rightly cautious, moves, as well as how it can ignore evidence to the detriment of patients for a long period of time.

The politics of Lyme includes some interesting facts:

• Unlike the case with other diseases, such as cancer, the diagnosis of Lyme depends on whether or not the doctor in question agrees with certain treatment protocols.

• Unlike the case with other diseases, the "cure" is defined in terms of how many antibiotics have been administered and for what length of time, rather than cessation of symptoms and absence of infection.

• Unlike the case with other diseases, the question of a Lyme diagnosis often rests solely upon the doctor's ability to make a clinical diagnosis (a return to the "old days" of medicine), instead of a reliance on empirical tests. Contemporary doctors are not trained for this and, in fact, are discouraged from trusting their clinical acumen.

• For any or all of the above reasons, Lyme diagnosis and treatment have caused medical professionals to take up arms against each other, each publicly hurling aspersions against the others' credibility and practices. These verbal attacks have been fired primarily from the purely academic researchers toward the clinician researchers and practitioners, whose work has been dismissed as "anecdotal" and "junk science."

Is this just another example of the age-old competition between the academicians, who enjoy the luxury of being more conservative because they are not dealing with patients daily, and the doctors in the trenches, who must treat sufferer after sufferer? Is it the snobbery of those who consider themselves "pure scientists" versus the "cowboys in the field" whose research may be privately funded? Perhaps. There is also the criticism that those associated with government and academic institutions must maintain lengthy time lines in research procedure in order to justify the much-needed allocations they receive.

All three points can be argued, and many of the more vociferous opponents on both sides suffer from what author Peter Senge, in his book *The Fifth Discipline*, calls one of the modern-day organizational learning disabilities: the "I am my position" identity, where a person stakes out a territory, identifies with it, and then defends it to the death—even in the face of contradictory evidence.

With Lyme disease, however, there is another factor involved. Because of the diversity of the disease and the lack of reliable empirical data, there is a great fear of personal liability.

FAULT, LIABILITY, AND RESPONSIBILITY

In a special exhibit presented at the National Museum of Health and Medicine in Washington, D.C., in November 1992, the question of medical ethics as it relates to human values and the complicity of doctors in Nazi experiments were highlighted. Entitled "The Value of the Human Being: Medicine in Germany, 1918–1945," the exhibit disturbed many in both the medical and the lay communities. The viewpoint was presented that during World War II, many doctors became agents of the state instead of advocates of the patient; they began viewing people as impersonal research statistics instead of individuals.

The exhibit further maintained that by joining the Nazi party, more than thirty-eight thousand doctors and scientists (almost half of Germany's total) were allowed to get research grants, receive promotions at universities, and take over the practices of the thousands of Jews who were no longer allowed to practice medicine.

The exhibit prompted Dr. James S. Todd, executive vice president of the American Medical Association, to comment in a *New York Times* article: "One of our biggest challenges today is balancing medicine and health against the resources available. But we have to strive to do this without forgetting about the patients we serve." Doctors, he said, have a special responsibility because people entrust them with their privacy as well as with their lives.

The politics of Lyme disease today can be likened somewhat to the mind-set of probably well-meaning physicians who got swept up in the Nazi regime. Struggling to support their families, continue their research, and maintain their career tracks, many unwittingly acted in passive complicity toward the deaths of millions.

Some may think this is too strong a statement—a totally inappropriate analogy. Yet when the most trusted professionals in a country—physicians—opt for reducing people and suffering to statistics because it allows them to comfortably maintain the status quo, as opposed to placing themselves and perhaps their careers on the line to relieve human suffering, isn't that reducing the value of a human being?

This is exactly what happens when a doctor refuses to listen to evidence of a disease—be it Lyme, AIDS, or cancer—because to diagnose and treat it might open him or her to question. This is exactly what happens when doctors who live in high-end suburban neighborhoods fight any acknowledgment of Lyme disease in their areas because they are afraid of their real estate values going down. And this is exactly what happens when otherwise bright and sincere doctors refuse to accept documentation of disease that is contrary to their "I am my position" stand, because to do so would mean admitting fallibility, even when human suffering is at stake.

I don't want to fall into the pit of indicting *all* doctors. There are many, many out there, God bless them, who do listen, and who do act as advocates for their patients at the risk of being considered out of the "mainstream." These men and women are true healers. Lyme disease, however, has caused many more to avoid some sticky issues, and sitting on the fence can cause a delay in diagnosis and therefore in treatment and possible eradication early on.

Another factor preventing doctors from dealing with Lyme is that we live in a litigious society. One cannot fault doctors for being cautious. It is also recognized that the practice of medicine is an *art* and not an exact science. But the "Amity-speak" at work here is: If I diagnose Lyme, I have to treat. If I treat and the patient doesn't respond well (or my peers object), I could be in trouble. Therefore, I won't diagnose.

This, unfortunately, is not an unusual position. And the one who pays is the patient, who can slip from a curable state into a debilitated and chronic condition.

INFORMED CONSENT AGREEMENTS

To respond to ailing patients with diffuse and Lyme-suspicious complaints, yet attempt to protect themselves, some doctors who treat the disease are taking a page out of the surgeon's guidebook and drawing up "informed consent" agreements.

Although viewed as impractical for a "normal" doctor-patient relationship, the informed consent agreement can be useful when dealing with a disease and treatment protocol that carry some controversy, according to Stephen Sepaniak, an attorney specializing in health and medicine in Lyme-endemic Morristown, New Jersey. And, if it encourages more doctors to deal with Lyme disease, such an agreement should be considered.

"One of the greatest areas of dispute between patients and physicians has to do with whether the physician disclosed to the patient all the risks of treatment, alternative forms of treatment, and even the risks of nontreatment. Clearly, these should be discussed," said Sepaniak. "When there are controversies surrounding treatment, as in Lyme disease, if I were a physician, I would spend a substantial amount of time discussing the different forms of treatment—reviewing the pros and cons of each regimen, and why one may be more appropriate than another. Only then would I give a patient my recommendation for a course of treatment and my reasons for that recommendation."

Some overcautious doctors videotape entire discussions and the patient's consent, but a written form is more standard. The paragraphs should include the benefits of the treatment, the risks, the alternative forms of treatment, and the risks of nontreatment. Then, the physician should outline his proposed course of action, with possible side effects, and sign the form, along with the patient.

"If a physician treats a patient negligently, he or she is still liable and no informed consent is going to provide blanket immunity," said Sepaniak, but the act of using an informed consent form forces the doctor to sit down and discuss, at length, the illness and the course of action. It takes some time, but it is a necessary expenditure of time that will benefit both the patient and the physician.

Educating and winning the proper attention of the country's populace is an important battle in the politics of diagnosing and treating Lyme. One would think that the education would come from the medical profession, but again, as with AIDS, it is the mass of Lyme sufferers and their loved ones who are leading the fight for recognition and treatment.

A GRASS ROOTS MOVEMENT

Dr. Vithal Shah practices in a rural town of one thousand residents in northern New Jersey. Out of that number, he is treating more than 120 people for Lyme disease. He knows the devastation it can wreak in a family because he and his wife, his children, and his mother-in-law, who came for a visit from India, all fell victim to it. He mounted an education campaign for his town that included bringing in some of the top researchers in the country to educate the other physicians and public health, school, and government officials to the spreading problem. "We have to take this to Washington," he says passionately. "The president has to hear how this illness is crippling the people of his nation."

■ Betty Gross, of Westchester, New York, never knows who is going to be on the other end of the telephone when she picks up one of her two lines each day from 8 A.M. to 4 P.M. The desperate calls for help come from as far away as Arizona and Oregon, from people searching for a physician who knows something about Lyme. The founder of the Lyme Support Group, the oldest and most activist organization in the country, the petite dynamo articulately and fervently intercedes for children who are suffering with Lyme when schools, teachers, physicians, and sometimes even parents ridicule, blame, or threaten them with punishment for "faking" pain, confusion, and inability to perform. She has initiated programs for doctors, legislators, school boards, and the court system. "This is an insidious and dangerous disease," she says. "We have to educate people—and physicians most of all!"

And in Coalinga, California, English teacher Laura Ames not only publishes a monthly newsletter titled *the ticked-off tract* but helps coordinate support group information, educational programs, and doctor referrals from as far away as Hawaii. Bitten by an infected tick in 1991, she began the informative publication out of "anger and frustration at not finding enough information at the patient level, and furor over what Lyme patients had to endure. Some patients, in wheelchairs because of Lyme, have to ask for a diagnosis of mental illness so they can get insurance coverage," she says. "We have to take an activist role in educating physicians and the public—and then make government listen, too!"

■ These stories are duplicated across the country. Faced with rejection, ignorance, and lack of treatment, men and women whose lives have been infected with Lyme become warriors in a battle for education and treatment. Some even leave their original professions behind in their fight for others' benefit.

The Lyme Disease Foundation was begun by businesswoman Karen Forschner, who contracted Lyme during her pregnancy with her son, Jamie. He was infected with the disease through the placenta and died after his first year of kindergarten from a series of malformations and complications arising from it. The foundation, run by Karen and her husband, Tom, has been responsible for international conferences, legislation, educational videos for both children and physicians, and continuing research and education on various aspects of the disease.

The Lyme Disease Network, based in East Brunswick, New Jersey, was begun by Carol and Bill Stolow after their three young daughters came down with Lyme and they had to fight for treatment on their behalf. Initially operating a hot line and educational service only in their home state, the network now helps coordinate information among support groups, doctors, researchers, and patients across the country, and provides an information line for doctors wishing to find out more about the disease.

People in several states have begun to learn about political maneuvering. We have seen the formation of coalitions, the appointing of the Governor's Council on Lyme Disease by New Jersey governor Jim Florio, and the growth of the activist group

VOICE (Victims of Insurance Company Exploitation), begun by Anne Ebert, whose children as well as herself are afflicted with Lyme, and dedicated to forcing insurance companies to live up to their contractual obligations and provide coverage for treatment (see chapter 17).

All of these groups notwithstanding, the recognition of Lyme disease as a potentially dangerous and debilitating illness begins with a recognition and acknowledgment that a problem does exist—as is illustrated by one of Dr. Masters's mental exercises. "Look around the room and for fifteen seconds memorize everything that's red," he says. "Now close your eyes. Tell me everything you saw in the room that was green. Chances are, you won't remember a thing. The eye only sees what the mind lets it. We have to let doctors realize that Lyme disease is out there so we can do something about it."

Recognition of Lyme begins with the symptoms, as varied and subjective as they may be, and then knowing where to go for help.

II.

SPECIAL AGES, SPECIAL PROBLEMS

■

"Knowledge is little; to know the right context is much; to know the right spot is everything."

—Hugo Von Hofmannsthal, Austrian poet and playwright

7.
The Young Child

Two-year-old Tommy had been considered mentally retarded almost since infancy. When a new pediatrician grew suspicious of this diagnosis during a patient history session with the parents, he ordered a new set of tests. Tommy's parents were both horrified and pleasantly stunned to find out that their son had Lyme disease, probably contracted when he was six months old and on a family vacation. After a course of aggressive antibiotic therapy, Tommy rebounded like the normal two-year-old he was.

■ Eight-year-old Jackie drove her teachers crazy with complaints. She had stomachaches, headaches, conjunctivitis, nausea, joint pain, blurry vision, and difficulty sitting still in class. The school nurse finally told her parents that they should consider psychological help for their obviously disturbed child. Four months and three doctors later, Jackie was diagnosed with Lyme disease and placed on antibiotics. Eighteen months later, she is on the soccer team, enjoys playing the piano, and is consistently on the honor roll.

■ Ten-year-old Jenna's Lyme disease followed a cycle similar to Jackie's, but she also lost the use of her right hand and arm. It took six months and five doctors before her parents found a doctor who believed that Jenna's symptoms had an organic, not a psychological, base, and who searched for the diagnosis. One evening, in the midst of a myriad of interviews and invasive tests, Jenna presented herself to her parents and tearfully cried, "I know what's wrong; I have AIDS and you just don't want to tell me!"

■ Fifty percent of all reported Lyme disease cases involve children under the age of twelve. Of that group, the largest percentage of victims are between the ages of one and five. If adults find respectful diagnosis and treatment difficult to obtain, they are even more elusive for young children who are dependent upon the adults in their world to listen, believe, understand, and then serve as tenacious advocates for them.

Some of the special challenges to diagnosing children ranging in age from infancy to eleven years old include:

• *They don't realize what is "normal."* Unlike adults, who have a track record of wellness, children, with their limited history and experience, may not even realize that everyone else walks around free of headache or of other symptoms that come and go.

• *They cannot always articulate symptoms.* This is particularly true in the prelanguage child, who must rely on the observations of the adults around him or her and their knowledge as to what is normal. Because so many children are also in day-care situations, there is a reliance on these caretakers to observe and note changes. Even the school-age child may have difficulty articulating a pain that waxes and wanes, periods of fatigue, or sensitivity to sound or touch.

• *They cannot remember sequences.* Children's frames of reference are such that if a hurt goes away they brush it from their minds and get on with life. If the pain returns, they may not be able to remember any sequential information that might provide some clue as to the pain's cause.

• *Getting someone to listen.* If adults find this aspect of disease reporting difficult, pity the poor child, who must compete in the adult world for attention to a stomachache, weak ankles, tingling in the fingers or face ("My face feels funny," said one little girl repeatedly to her dad. "Your face *looks* funny," he would lovingly reply. Unfortunately, she was trying to tell him she was feeling tingling—a neurological symptom), and changes in sleep or personal patterns. (How many well-meaning parents crack down on television watching, play activities, and snacks when confronted with a child who complains that he can't sleep at night, has diarrhea, or is tired in school?)

• *Being believed.* More often than not, the children who complain of a kaleidoscope of aches are told they have growing pains, are just trying to get attention, are attempting to get out of school/homework/chores, are malingering, or simply are faking it.

In the popular movie *Ferris Bueller's Day Off,* the following advice is sagely given: "Don't overfake; it will get you a trip to the pediatrician and that's worse!" Dr. Louis Corsaro, a pediatrician and father of eight who practices in the hyperendemic area of Westchester County, New York, firmly believes the film's advice mirrors reality, and that more parents, teachers, and doctors need to listen to the young child who is attempting to convey a message of illness, particularly if something like Lyme disease is a possibility.

"Children don't lie when it comes to aches and pains, and they don't exaggerate," he said. "It should be easy to tell when a child is really ill because they only have two speeds—sleep and fast. As a pediatrician in an area where I've handled more than twelve hundred cases of Lyme—three hundred and fifty of those in the chronic stage—there is no question in my mind that if a diagnosis is made early, short-term antibiotics are effective. But if children are dismissed as complainers, if there is a delay in focusing on the symptoms that are being presented—particularly if one is living in an area where Lyme is endemic—the child can go into a chronic stage, which is much more difficult to treat."

Add to the physical derailment the psychological manifestations that accompany Lyme, and you have children who are being told that their pains are all in their heads or who are suddenly labeled as learning disabled or victims of attention deficit disorder (ADD) and are funneled into neatly labeled classes and categories where they languish or continue their deterioration.

The best prevention is knowing what to look for and how to get help.

CHILDREN AND SYMPTOMS

Dr. Dorothy Pietrucha's office is in an unprepossessing white expanded ranch not far from the Garden State Parkway in Neptune, New Jersey—one of the epidemic Lyme centers for the country. Parents bring their children from as far away as California, Florida, Minnesota, and Virginia to see this pediatric neurologist who, as a medical adviser to both the Prevent Lyme Foundation and the Lyme Disease Foundation and director of the Division of Pediatric Neurology at Jersey Shore Medical Center, has documented and treated more than a thousand cases of pediatric Lyme, and tenaciously fights for her patients.

She presents a sensible picture: trademark suit with stock tie blouse, sensible shoes, and fresh-scrubbed face. She speaks quickly and confidently—gently to the children, forcefully when discussing how the politics of Lyme is promoting late diagnosis and its long-term effects on children, and passionately when arguing over treatment standards. Her presentations at both national and international Lyme conferences have opened many doctors' eyes to the numbers of children being affected by this disease.

"Over the past nine years, I have had to treat more than three hundred children for Lyme disease in the hospital because they had significant neurologic manifestations of the disease or, in a minority of cases, an arthritis necessitating hospitalization for intravenous antibiotics. Many of these children are not diagnosed initially because their complaints are vague and are thought to be functional. I have treated a patient who has been sick for five years. Others were sick three and four years before being diagnosed.

"I have seen children develop neurologic symptoms within a few weeks after a tick bite, while others will not develop the symptoms for a year or more. Less than fifty percent of the children even remember being bitten by a tick, and even a smaller percentage than that remember any ECM rash," she said.

"One of the telltale situations is that the parents recall the children having a flulike illness that preceded their developing these rather persistent symptoms. Usually, that flulike illness will occur six weeks or more after the tick bite or the exposure to the ticks. Many parents claim that after this 'flulike' illness, the child was never well again."

The symptoms that children experience parallel those for adults, with emphasis on:

- Headache (more than 90 percent complain of this; they usually do not respond to over-the-counter analgesics)
- Sensitivity to light
- Dizziness
- Stiff neck
- Backache
- Sleepiness
- Memory problems

- Difficulty concentrating
- Stomach pain (50 percent complain of this; a significant percentage may also have an ulcer)
- Mood swings and irritability (even in very young children)
- Chest pain (70 percent complained of this)
- Joint pain (primarily knees, wrists, and ankles)
- Sore throats ("The worst sore throat ever!" is a common complaint)
- Heart palpitations
- Tingling or numbness
- Rashes that come and go
- Letter and number reversals
- Pain caused by swelling of the optic nerve
- Weakness in a limb
- Bell's palsy

Children with central or peripheral nervous system involvement may also have wake-sleep disturbances, difficulty concentrating, episodes of disorientation, difficulty spelling words they could spell before the illness, and difficulty learning new material.

In attempting to describe symptoms, kids will be very specific—"my left knee" or "a headache at the front of my head." This type of complaint deserves attention.

It is easy to see from this varied list why parents and teachers may be skeptical at first when presented with continual complaints, but that, in itself, should be a red flag to pay attention.

THE "FAKING IT" MYTH

Despite such dismissal by some teachers and doctors, children do not fake Lyme disease or its symptoms. The reason is simple. To do so would take too great a toll on the child, even if he or she could conceive and carry off such a plan.

"Kids ask why I've been so sick and I said, 'Lyme disease,' " said Billy. "They say, 'Lyme disease! Get away from me.' They think they can catch it and they won't play with me and they leave me out of things."

A major portion of a child's life is spent involved with school and friends. Yes, a child can fake one stomachache to get out of a math test. But children do not fake continually changing symptoms because the result may be the loss of social contact, being left behind in school, unpleasant medical treatment, and an inability to participate in previously enjoyed sports and activities.

No child would rather be declared chronically ill and have to do schoolwork at home, all by himself, for days on end. No child is going to give up Scouts, teams, field trips, overnights, parties, and music, dance, or riding lessons that are enjoyed. And no child can keep a charade going for the length of time the symptoms last in patients with Lyme.

"When Jenna said she couldn't use her arm and hand, my husband and I watched her at a friend's birthday party," said Ginny. "We thought maybe she'd forget and reach for something. But what we saw was a little girl trying desperately to enjoy the party and almost absentmindedly holding her numb arm with her good hand. That really convinced us."

Nobody knows a child like a parent does. Better than any doctor, teacher, or friend, a parent can tell when a child "isn't right," despite tests to the contrary. It is that inside knowledge regarding a child that places a parent in a position to be that child's advocate. And this is a very necessary position.

PARENTS AS ADVOCATES

When my son was first ill and we were going through the myriad tests to eliminate other problems, I quickly found that unless one spoke in a very insistent voice, it was easy to be relegated to a place in the woodwork. One lab did tests for our particular medical group, but tests were read only once a week because that was the group's day. Meanwhile, my child was getting worse on a daily basis.

It was absurd to wait a week for test results that were sitting on a desk, test results that would help determine the next step to my son's wellness. I expressed that feeling very clearly to the doctor and volunteered to pick up the tests and deliver them myself if he couldn't handle getting to the lab. We had the results read the following day and continued the process. My son could never have accomplished this on his own behalf. The complacency that sets in when routines are followed leads people to ignore desperate situations.

Growing up in a European-type household did not prepare me for having to fight authority figures, but when the realization dawned that the only thing standing between my child's life and possible death was me, I developed a different attitude. And *that* is what each of us must do for our children, whether we suspect they have Lyme disease or another difficult illness.

No longer do I sit back meekly and accept others' rules if they infringe on my son's progress. No longer do I sit passively in conferences and accept what "knowledgeable" educators, doctors, and counselors say as gospel. I don't care if they are experts in their respective fields; I am an expert when it comes to my children. I like to think that I am courteous, but make no mistake—I am firm. After all, no matter the ages of the children, their voices just don't command the attention an adult's does, and it is the loud and insistent voice that gets action.

"You have to be an advocate for your child," agrees Carol Stolow, who with her husband, Bill, founded the Lyme Disease Network after her three daughters contracted Lyme. "Sometimes you have to take on the doctors, take on the school and teachers—everyone who's telling you what they think is wrong with your child. Sometimes they're looking for an easy 'out'; sometimes there's a different agenda. But your child needs to have representation in all of these arenas by someone who believes in and can fight for his or her rights."

Unfortunately, with Lyme, that advocacy is becoming important even in one's own household. Sometimes other family members doubt the diagnosis and question the child's motives in "acting sick." In a scattering of extreme cases, the controversy over a Lyme diagnosis and treatment is being used as a weapon in divorce cases, with one partner charging that the other is neurotically insisting a child is sick when he or she isn't and is therefore an unfit parent.

But nowhere does the child need an advocate more than at school, where many teachers and administrators are still ignorant regarding the disease and its effects on children.

DEALING WITH SCHOOLS

Education is the best defense against Lyme disease, and one of the more important groups of people to educate is the educators—those individuals who see our children for a longer period of time than a parent does on any given school day. For it is in the classroom, and under stress, that Lyme symptoms will most commonly be apparent.

"I told the teacher I had a really bad headache at the front of my head," said eleven-year-old Tara. "She said, 'Oh, you have headaches every day. Can't you skip it today?' "

Nine-year-old Bill kept falling down during soccer practice. When he complained that his joints had been hurting and his ankles were weak, the coach scolded him for being a "weenie" and directed, "Play with pain. That's what the professionals do!"

Tina had been a strong A/B student all through her six years of school. Then, in seventh grade, her schoolwork began falling off, particularly math and Spanish. She complained of headaches and could barely stay awake in class. When she told her teachers that she was having trouble concentrating, they told her parents that Tina was becoming learning disabled and recommended both special-ed classes and a psychiatrist to help with her attention deficit disorder. Fortunately, Tina's doctor listened carefully and decided to test for Lyme disease. Tina's serology was positive, probably the result of a tick bite when visiting her cousins in California before school began.

▪ For children, success in school is equated with success in life because school is, after all, their full-time job. When a child is infected with Lyme disease, physical symptoms impede the natural learning processes, and the child's credibility with the adults in charge becomes shaky. This further erodes the child's self-esteem for future performance.

Adding to the child's frustration and downward spiral are absences from school, resulting in pressure to catch up; isolation from or rejection by friends; and the frustration of attempting to learn when impaired memory and concentration, and other physical ailments, block learning receptors. It is important for educators to recognize a tick and know how to remove it, but it is not enough to merely stop there. Teachers and administrators need to be just as informed as physicians in recognizing the physical and psychological presentations of Lyme that they may see in the classroom.

This is a very real problem for many school districts, says John Staryak, supervisor of guidance services for the Jackson Township school district in New Jersey. At any given time, 15 to 20 percent of his student population can be down with Lyme disease. In most districts, when 30 percent of a school population has an illness, they close the schools.

"You can walk through the halls and look in classrooms,

and you'll see kids with their heads down on the desks. These kids have Lyme disease, and it's become so common that the teachers and other kids in the class just accommodate it," says the tall, sandy-haired, former middle school teacher. "Unfortunately, this illness is impacting on the classroom, on the material, and on how teachers function in the class. I see us as having to deal with a whole different classification of learning-disabled student—they fall somewhere between chronically ill and learning impaired. And teachers need to have more in-services regarding the recognition of Lyme symptoms because we can't uniformly classify these students as perceptually impaired.

"Most of what the teachers see are fatigue (our teachers let the kids put their heads down), headaches, and short-term memory loss. This is especially troublesome in math, where if you don't get the first concept, you can't get the next, which builds on it. Foreign language, too, uses the building block concept and is a particular problem for kids with Lyme. History and English seem to be all right, if the kid can get a grasp of it when she is feeling well."

In Jackson, as in a number of school systems across the country, the schools have to provide an additional learning and support program after school called "Supplemental." With Supplemental, a new contingent of teachers arrives to tutor those kids who are having difficulties with their regular schoolwork due to absences and Lyme disease.

Staryak dynamically asserts that this is only a beginning, because the whole approach to learning and student management is going to have to change as well to deal with the effects of this spreading illness.

"First, there *has* to be communication between the parents and the school. We—the counselor, nurse, and guidance department—need to know up front that the child has Lyme so we can get it out to the teachers involved.

"Secondly, we have to provide more in-servicing for the teachers on the predictable effects of Lyme disease; what to do and what not to do, as well as some strategies for helping these kids. It's not enough to rattle off a list of symptoms. The individual institutions, as much as possible, have to break the 'tyranny of the textbook' mold. We have to look at students in a more individualistic and holistic way, with more attention paid to the pace of the individual than to the pace of the class.

"Thirdly, we need an alternative means of assessment for these students," said Staryak intently. "The easiest tests to correct are true-false tests, but this is where portfolio and contract learning come in. The Lyme disease student has difficulty storing and processing information. We need to teach students how to *manage* information, where to find and store it; in other words, the *process*, not the product, becomes the important thing. And that will be a very useful thing to teach all students."

Staryak said he realizes that these ideas would demand that teachers take the classical structure of a classroom and throw it out the window, but the impact of Lyme students and others with temporary or permanent disabilities is such that flexibility is going to be demanded on an increasing basis.

Under current federal and state regulations, children with chronic illness can receive an individualized educational program (IEP) that will accommodate their special needs. For Lyme patients, this may include at-home tutoring, a shorter school day, or supplemental instruction at the school. It is important to find out what is available in your particular school district that will assist your child in obtaining a good education. (After all, you *are* paying for it, whether through taxes or tuition.)

If the teachers in your child's school are unfamiliar with Lyme disease, you would be providing a major service by initiating a special information session through a local support group, hospital, public health agency, or informed doctor who is dealing with Lyme.

After all the pain, doubts, fears, and suffering children with Lyme have to go through, they need all the informed support possible in order to maintain a normal life. And those children in the adolescent-to-teenage range have an additional set of problems with which to cope.

8.
The Teenager

During the spring of his fifteenth year, my son Christopher was on his school's track and field team, learning to pole-vault, running three miles a day while listening to Air Force and Naval Academy motivational tapes, and actively participating in school projects. An honor student since elementary school, he was on the advanced track in both math and science in a rigorous Northeastern private school. His easygoing manner and quick wit attracted numerous friends, and his plans for the next year included fulfilling a lifelong ambition—working toward his pilot's license, having already obtained his ham radio license the previous year.

During the summer, he went to the family pediatrician with several raised rashes on his legs and arms. The doctor diagnosed "summer rashes" and prescribed cortisone cream. A month later, Chris's glands were swollen, his throat sore, and his joints achy. The pediatrician treated him for mononucleosis and warned that it would take months to get over its effects.

That fall, Chris's grades began to slip. He grew alternately irritable and lethargic. He began to have trouble sleeping and felt dizzy and achy. He refrained from participating in school activities and stopped his trademark voracious reading. He broke up with his girlfriend and walked out on an aptitude test—something he normally found pleasantly challenging. When a school counselor suggested that Chris drop to a lower track in math and science, it was decided that all he needed was more discipline and less party time.

By Christmas, Chris was experiencing episodes of tremors, wherein his body would shake and twitch uncontrollably. The dizziness and pressure in his head were almost constant now. The pediatrician, after reviewing negative tests for brain tumors and MS, decided that Chris's cerebellum—the center of balance—was inflamed and prescribed Dramamine. Another month, four more doctors, and thousands of dollars in diagnostic tests later, the only suggestions from specialists were for Chris to see a psychiatrist for his increasing depression, irritability, lack of concentration, and episodes of tremors. School officials decided Chris must be on drugs. This "diagnosis" was proven false through a thorough drug screening.

Then, on Super Bowl Sunday, while at the home of good friends and in the midst of a congenial get-together, Chris had an episode of tremors that lasted two hours. By this time, I had read enough information on Lyme disease to demand the name of a Lyme specialist, despite several doctors' protests.

In the spring of his sixteenth year, Chris completed his second month of intravenous therapy, which had relieved most of his symptoms. After finishing the intravenous antibiotics, he was put on oral antibiotics following a relapse that brought back all of the original symptoms, including the tremors. He could not participate in sports; he had to drop chemistry, drop down a track in math, and anticipated repeating Spanish, because these three subjects depend on sequential learning—something of which he was incapable during the fall and winter. Despite the fact that he was dying to get his learner's permit to drive a car, he postponed that until he was confident that the tremors and dizziness were gone for good.

Now, in the winter of his seventeenth year, Chris is hopeful that he has beaten the spirochete but is worried about relapsing again. After ten months of antibiotics, he stopped taking them and, with a doctor's help, began to rehabilitate his body through nutrition, supplements, and exercise. Some days are very good and some days are bad.

On a bad day, he finds it difficult to get up from the couch to answer the telephone, and depression is always a step away. On a good day, he tends to overdo it in order to make up for all the days of feeling lousy—which tends to backfire. Getting his pilot's license is on the back burner. His short-term goal is simple: "I just look forward to feeling normal again. I've forgotten what that's like."

■ Although teens can usually articulate symptoms, there are so many other psychological and physiological processes going on during adolescence that doctors tend to look past the presenting symptoms for something more developmentally oriented—rebellion, raging hormones, drug abuse, and immaturity. Because of this, a significant percentage of teenage Lyme victims go undiagnosed until the condition is so severe that the child requires hospitalization, or until so many systems of the body are degenerating that serious attention is finally given.

Ask any adult if she or he would like to be fifteen again, and chances are the emphatic answer will be "No way!" Even at its best, adolescence is a pain for all concerned. There are issues of separation from parents, which touch off various forms of rebellion, the search for an identity and independence, and the exploration of new behaviors. There are social issues involving interaction with various hierarchies of society, including members of the opposite sex, and social choices regarding such things as alcohol, drugs, and sexual experimentation. And there are career goals and issues that propel the teen through a myriad of tests, options, and decisions.

Normal teens can experience mood swings, irritability, raging hormones that manifest in headaches, stress presenting as stomachaches, and a desire for individualization that is noticeable when they exhibit antisocial behavior around their parents.

Throw in a couple of curves like drug and alcohol experimentation, and is it any wonder that—without the benefit of seeing the rash (and not many parents see their teens' bodies unclothed)—parents, teachers, and doctors may have difficulty distinguishing where normal teenage angst ends and Lyme disease begins?

WHAT'S WRONG WITH THIS KID?

Fourteen-year-old Todd was found wandering the halls of the school. He received detentions for being "rebellious." The vice principal didn't believe him when, scared and upset, Todd told him he got lost.

Seventeen-year-old Wendy began falling down at school. Her lethargy, dropping grades, and inability to concentrate led the school counselor to recommend discipline for drug use.

Sixteen-year-old Jamie was becoming more and more frightened. Always a good student, his scores suddenly plunged in math, and he struggled in language arts. He realized that he was reversing numbers, in addition to having to deal with a constant headache and fatigue.

■ Unfortunately, in today's society, drug abuse is a legitimate concern when a teen's behavior and school performance change for the worse. This is probably the only age group where the first differential diagnosis that pops into mind is drug abuse, and so it must be ruled out before any credibility is given to any other diagnosis.

It doesn't make any sense to fight doing a drug screen. In

fact, I would insist on it. The screen is a simple, noninvasive test. If it is positive, then you know you have one major problem to deal with; if it is negative, it just reaffirms that something else is wrong.

Apart from a drug screen, how can a parent, doctor, or educator distinguish between the normal teen problems and signs of Lyme?

"Look for chronicity," says Dr. Pietrucha. "This is where the patient history is most important. This is a child who is suddenly always sick. It is a teenager's nature to complain about a lot of things, but when you get right down to it, they go to school and get their work done.

"With Lyme, these kids become so unwell that they aren't capable of getting their work done, no matter what you say."

Drs. Fallon and Corsaro also recommend that you look for cognitive problems, including:

- Memory loss
- Disorientation
- Sudden onset of dyslexic tendencies
- Difficulty concentrating
- Sleep disturbances (insomnia; lethargy and sleepiness)

In addition, look for emotional instability such as overreactions and crying easily or suddenly. In reviewing dropped grades, pinpoint which subjects are plunging. If they are math, foreign languages, and science (such as chemistry), this is indicative of short-term memory and other cognitive problems.

Teens who are experimenting with drugs generally have a close circle of friends who are also involved. Teens who are infected with Lyme don't have the energy, stamina, or inclination to get together with friends.

Lyme presents the teen with frustrating problems that impinge on the normal issues of separation, identity, socialization, and goal setting. At a time when they are attempting to break away, they suddenly find themselves in a more dependent position because of their sickness and increasing psychological symptoms. At a time when they are trying to forge an identity, they are forced to defend their credibility if their symptoms are unbelieved, to the point of self-doubt and plummeting self-esteem. At a time when they should be learning new socialization patterns, the unpredictability of Lyme continually impedes their participation in social gatherings, commitments, and relationships. And at a time when they would normally be setting life and work goals, they are physically and emotionally restricted to fighting simply for wellness and perhaps watching certain dreams fade into the background.

Add to this the normal stresses of schoolwork and psychosocial development and you have a formula for a very unhappy camper.

If adults face ignorance about Lyme in the workplace and the medical field, teens don't fare much better. Despite the fact that they would normally rather have people think they hatched from eggs fully formed than admit they have parents who care, the teen Lyme patient, as well as the younger child, needs an advocate to represent him or her to those who unknowingly or uncaringly denigrate his or her rights and condition.

Then there are arrogant administrators such as the one who (though fully informed of fifteen-year-old Michael's condition and able to *see* he had an intravenous catheter in his arm) delivered the following "hit-and-run" message in the school hall before he strode on, leaving the struggling teenager devastated: "You know, I'm tired of you acting sick. You should be well by now!"

Or inconsiderate counselors like the one who commented to a seventeen-year-old Lyme patient, "Well, now that you're learning disabled, I guess you'll be looking into easy jobs instead of applying to college, huh?"

Or well-meaning, overachieving fathers like the one who refused to let the school classify his daughter as chronically ill because he thought it would look bad on her college applications.

College applications *are* a very real worry for many teens with Lyme, but hope and understanding are definitely at the end of the tunnel, as the effects of Lyme disease are being recognized by some of the country's major institutions.

THE COLLEGE APPLICATION DILEMMA

Since it is generally acknowledged that the junior year in high school is of utmost importance in the college application procedure, the worst-case scenario for a teen would then be to contract Lyme prior to the junior year and suffer through the year undiagnosed, or in the early stages of treatment.

Loss of time in school plus the cumulative physical and psychological effects of undiagnosed or chronic Lyme can add up to a year that is a washout in terms of grades and activities. And that's if the child is able to remain in school at all. There are many who have had to study at home on a long-term basis because they could not handle the day's unrelenting schedules.

Then too, there is the concern over taking the SATs—that standard yardstick used by most colleges in the admission process. Lyme disease certainly affects test-taking skills as much as it affects overall school performance. Because of the spread of Lyme disease, the Educational Testing Service, in Princeton, New Jersey, has made available an untimed SAT for which students can make application with supportive evidence from their doctors.

Experienced physicians such as Corsaro and Pietrucha also become an integral part of their student-patients' college application procedures by writing letters of recommendation explaining the extenuating circumstances surrounding the students' records.

These letters usually point out that the student was chronically ill during high school and for that reason grades may not have been up to what they would normally have been. They maintain that the student is presently improved and deserves the opportunity to study and get as complete an education as he or she desires.

"I've now had patients who have finished college and their grades and performance in college were considerably better than in high school," said Pietrucha. "They seem to be sickest during their high school years but then get on top of it. I'm optimistic that if a student gets treatment, even if he or she has some rough years, they can pursue a college education and further degrees if that's what they want."

College and tests aside, in the "black or white" world of teenagers, just getting through the disease is a major accomplishment. How do teens successfully cope? With a new awareness of their own mortality.

GETTING THROUGH IT—A NEW AWARENESS

Most of the kids Abby's age talk about rock stars, school tests, shopping malls, and the boys in class. Fourteen-year-old Abby's conversation is dotted with terms such as "spirochetes," "white-cell counts," "remitting and relapsing," and "encephalopathy." Her eyes fill with tears when she stops to think of how lonely she is, unable to join the other girls in normal social activities. Her Lyme went undiagnosed for more than two years. She is now into her tenth month of treatment, and her big goal in life is to be able to attend high school like a normal teenager.

"I feel like I am so far behind all the kids I used to hang out with," she says. "They are moving forward, making plans, *doing* things. I feel like a little kid, tied to medicines and my mommy. I don't want to live the rest of my life like this."

Chronic illness of any kind must be terribly frustrating. When it hits young people it carries a double whammy because until a cure is developed, the roller coaster of illness becomes a way of life.

Some doctors feel that teenage boys seem to cope better with Lyme disease by incorporating the necessary routines into their schedules and displaying a more optimistic attitude regarding wellness than some girls, who have tried to take overdoses of sleeping pills to end the pain. On occasion, the frustration over the needless intensity of the illness due to lack of knowledge and diagnosis of Lyme overtakes some teens, who exhibit a rage response. These are usually isolated instances, however. If this type of reaction becomes part of the everyday pattern, then it would be wise to seek counseling for that child.

Actually, for those who are in the chronic stage of Lyme, counseling can provide many benefits, if only to help the teen deal with a long-term illness and assure him or her that he or she is not going crazy.

The teens themselves find various methods of getting through the tedium of feeling unwell, stymied activities, and academic struggles.

"Don't doubt yourself," says Kelly, sixteen. "And try not to let doctors bully you into doubting yourself. Remember, there are still a few good doctors who will try their best to find a cure for you."

Seventeen-year-old Chris recommends that teens focus on short-term goals. "Find something to look forward to—a concert, a party, getting together with a friend you haven't seen in a long time—something that you can set your mind on when your body is feeling lousy. Also, it helps to have an outlet for those feelings of frustration. I took up the drums and it really helps; it's also good exercise and I feel better after I've played."

"Try to keep to as normal a routine as possible," says Jeremy, fifteen. "I know some kids with Lyme find it hard to even get out of bed, but it's important to try to do all the regular things. I like to take a walk around the block and look at the people and things around me."

All the teens I spoke to agree that keeping in touch with friends is very important, even during those times that they felt the worst. It helped to focus their attention on something outside themselves and their aches and pains.

One word of caution, however. With chronic or late-stage Lyme there are so many days when the teen feels crummy that on those few days when the symptoms blend into the background, the child wants to pour all of his or her energy into activities in a seemingly frantic attempt to make up for lost time. This can lead to overexertion, which inevitably results in a physical and emotional "crash" afterward. It is difficult for a parent to apply the "brakes," so to speak, particularly when you empathize with your child's desire to be "normal," but it is advisable.

One by-product of teenage Lyme is that the youngsters involved develop an awareness of their own mortality that is not common in most kids their age.

"I think I'm more careful when I drive, and I tend to look out for the other kids I'm with," says Jean, seventeen and a Lyme patient for two years. "Sometimes I feel more like their mother than their friend, but I know I can die. I don't think I'm immortal. I came too close to dying or at least feeling like I was going to die, with Lyme. Maybe, after I'm cured, I'll forget these feelings, but for right now, I try to appreciate the good moments."

■ It is disturbing when children and teens contract Lyme and go undiagnosed. It is perhaps also frustrating and guilt-inspiring when an infected mother is not recognized as having Lyme, goes untreated, and passes that disease on to her unborn child.

9.
The Pregnant Woman

When a pregnant woman contracts Lyme disease, not only does she run the risk of progressively debilitating symptoms that parallel progressive infection, so does her unborn baby. Medical documentation indicates that there is a transfer of the spirochetes from the mother's body through the placenta to the fetus.

This in utero infection by the Lyme organism can result in stillbirth, spontaneous abortion, and damage to the brain, heart, liver, and other organs. Or it can result in the newborn's living a life of chronic illness that baffles pediatricians, puts stress on the family, and prevents the child from growing, thriving, and socializing within the normal parameters of development.

A FAMILY ILLNESS

Lynn had everything going for her when she was bitten by an infected tick on vacation during the summer of 1983. She held a high-powered job as a financial analyst in New York City, she was engaged to be married, and her outgoing nature kept her in a whirl of outdoor and social activities. By her September wedding date, two months later, she had been treated for a virulent "flu," had been diagnosed as having shoulder problems, and underwent an appendectomy. Four months later, another doctor said she had thyroid problems, depression, and menstrual irregularities.

By September of 1984, she was so chronically ill that she had to give up her job.

Not only did this put a strain on her new marriage, but during her pregnancy a year later she experienced increasingly varied symptoms, culminating in a neurological stroke. At least baby Lauren was healthy, she thought desperately, when she was told in the delivery room that the Apgar score was perfect.

That jubilation lasted only four months, however, because the infant soon developed ring rashes all over her ankles. At five months, she began experiencing a series of chronic ear infections, and by seventeen months she suffered from severe pneumonia. Repeated trips to pediatricians and specialists could not uncover the causes of the continual stomach pains, sore throats, recurring fevers, and chronic illness.

Although Lynn herself was continually sick, she tried to keep a low profile on her own aches and pains as she tended her sick child and nursed the hope that the new child she was carrying would be born in good health. But this second pregnancy only exacerbated her varied symptoms and led her to be hospitalized at New York City's Columbia Presbyterian Hospital for a repeated series of tests that kept proving negative.

Jack was born five weeks premature and seemed to be ill from the beginning. He cried fourteen hours a day, gained very little weight, suffered from the same upper respiratory problems as his sister, and screamed when he urinated.

As Lynn saw both her children struggle to survive, and a plethora of doctors pass them around, a rage built inside that motivated her to begin taking medical courses at the local university. But the knowledge that the courses brought could not stop her own deterioration, which led to surgery for damage to her liver and pancreas. From 1990 to 1992, she made the rounds of doctors who were looking for autoimmune disorders, doctors who inspired her to examine her life for illness-oriented behaviors, and doctors who told her that her problems and those of her children were all in her head.

Then, in January of 1992, after she and her children suffered agonizing bouts of "flu," chicken pox, and heart problems, Lynn tested positive for Lyme disease. Shortly thereafter, her children were diagnosed with congenital Lyme. All began treatment.

Today, Lauren has an abnormal EEG that indicates temporal lobe seizure disorder, an abnormal MRI, and hyperactivity disorders. Jack suffers from sensory deficiencies, migrating pain, and attention deficit disorders aggravated by the Lyme.

And Lynn, in order to help other families, educate doctors, and assist in finding a cure for the ailment that now infects eleven of her family members and eighteen of her immediate neighbors, established the Prevent Lyme Foundation. Its primary areas of research are entomological studies at Rutgers University, PCR studies at Fox Chase in Philadelphia, and neuropsychiatric studies at New York Psychiatric Hospital. In addition, the foundation has put together educational programs for schools, sponsored a Lyme awareness march across the state of New Jersey, established a professional Lyme publication for physicians, and is organizing family counseling support services.

"We have to prevent the late diagnosis of Lyme and make sure that all pregnant women who suspect they have Lyme disease get to knowledgeable doctors who will treat them aggressively to prevent what happened to my children," says Lynn, an intensely articulate and attractive brunette whose eyes widen behind slightly oversized glasses.

"I keep telling myself that we'll beat this thing," she said, her eyes filling. "I made a promise to myself. I have to do this for my son, who wakes up in the middle of the night and cries to please make the pain go away. I have to do this for my daughter, whose fists I have to hold as she's crying and trying to hit me in a confused and painful rage. And also for my father, who at age fifty-seven has been told he has permanent brain damage now because of Lyme and that if it had been diagnosed five years ago, he wouldn't have this.

"People have to hear the true story of what Lyme disease can do to your life and the lives of those you love. The Prevent Lyme Foundation is trying to tell this story through research and education."

■ The studies done on pregnancy and Lyme disease are few and far between. According to Dr. Louis Bracero, associate professor of obstetrics and gynecology at New York Medical College, Lyme disease follows the pattern of other spirochetal illnesses that are contracted via the placenta during pregnancy. Lyme spirochetes have been found in the liver, heart, and other organs of babies who were born to women with Lyme and who died. A study by Dr. Alan MacDonald, of Southampton Hospital, in New York, revealed that Lyme disease acquired in utero may result in fetal death either in utero or shortly after birth. He also discovered that tissue inflammation was not seen in fetuses that acquired Lyme disease through the placenta, and that in all but one of the cases where the Lyme organism was identified in the placenta or the fetal tissues, the maternal blood had no evidence of antibodies to the Lyme bacteria.

Continuing research regarding transplacental Lyme is being undertaken by the Lyme Disease Foundation in Tolland, Connecticut, which examines placentas for evidence of spirochetes, but many more studies are needed.

There is a concern among pregnant women who have tested positive for Lyme in the past, successfully completed treatment, and remain asymptomatic that their babies still might acquire Lyme in utero. Some have even expressed confusion over whether their pregnancies should be terminated.

Drs. Len Sigal and Ana Fernandez, of the Lyme Disease Center, Robert Wood Johnson Medical School, feel that while

pregnancy complicated by Lyme disease should not be terminated, treatment of the mother's Lyme should be undertaken
immediately to prevent ensuing complications. This view is also
held by experts across the country, including Dr. Paul Lavoie,
of Pacific Presbyterian Medical Center in San Francisco, who
first identified Lyme arthritis in California in 1975 and skin
inflammation linked to chronic Lyme. Dr. Lavoie, who authored
the Lyme disease section of *Conn's Current Therapy*, the treatment "bible" of physicians, says that the likelihood that the
fetus will be infected through the placenta is highest early in the
disease, when it is being quickly disseminated by the blood. For
this reason, a pregnant woman who contracts Lyme, particularly
during the first trimester of pregnancy, should be treated aggressively with antibiotics. There is a risk throughout the entire
pregnancy, however, that the mother will pass the spirochetal
infection to her unborn infant, and Lavoie also advises that
treatment would seem to be indicated throughout the pregnancy
for the best protection for the baby.

While this would seem to be fairly straightforward advice
regarding pregnancy and Lyme, the obstacle once again is diagnosis, and pregnant women face nearly as much prejudice as do
teenagers.

"OH, YOU'RE JUST PREGNANT!"

Being a mother is everything to Diane, who lives in Pennsylvania.
"My kids are my life," cheerfully states this mother of four with
another on the way. This, her fifth pregnancy, has brought about
a whole set of problems and prejudices, however, that Diane
never expected to encounter.

She doesn't remember a tick bite, but she distinctly remembers the beginning of her symptoms early in her pregnancy.

First came the stiff neck, swollen glands, lump in her throat, headaches, and incredible fatigue. By the end of June (two months into the pregnancy), she had pain in her chest when she took a breath. When she told her obstetrician, he said, "You're pregnant. Pregnant women are supposed to get aches and pains." After the chest pains, he blamed her aches on a lack of sleep and prescribed Tylenol with codeine. Despite the fact that she protested that she knew what the aches of pregnancy were and this was different, that she didn't feel "right," she was told it was because of her condition.

A month later, while on vacation, she had to be rushed to a hospital emergency room with what she thought was a heart attack. Tests revealed nothing. Maybe it was bronchitis, the doctors suggested.

Ensuing symptoms included chills (during warm weather), continued chest pain, blurred vision, light-headedness, and hypersensitivity of her legs, back, and head. Diane tried to explain this to her doctor again—and to a couple of specialists along the way. She was told, "Go home and do Lamaze breathing and everything will be fine."

By this time she had heard of Lyme disease, and she requested information on it. "Oh, it's the 'in' disease to have right now. Don't worry about it," said the doctor.

She thought her problems were over when she was finally put in touch with a doctor who did see Lyme cases, but she was told that despite the fact that he suspected Lyme, he wouldn't treat pregnant women. Seeking help from the University of Pennsylvania, she was told that they would treat her only if she would transfer all of her records to them and have her baby there. Though she felt she couldn't do that, they gave her two weeks' worth of antibiotics, which she took.

"For five days I felt normal," she says. "Then I got a burning in my joints and the pain in my head came back. I went to a rheumatologist, who would not even test me for Lyme because he said that if I had been on antibiotics for two weeks I was cured.

"At seven months pregnant, I'm still not feeling good. I get strange headaches, feel out of it. The pain has been so horrible that I've even packed my head in ice to try and stop it. Nothing works, and no one will treat me. They say to come back after I give birth if I still have a problem. I went to a neurologist who told me I'd feel better after the baby was born. I was worried about the baby so I went to a perinatalogist, who checked and said the baby looks okay but is several weeks behind in developing.

"I'm very worried, with all the evidence of stillbirths and miscarriages. Every doctor has blamed my pregnancy and the fact that it is my fifth child," says Diane heatedly. "I got so tired of hearing it, I wanted to punch them! Believe me, I'm happy to be pregnant—I wanted this—but what I'm feeling isn't pregnancy. It's different, and when I feel the pains, I have to wonder, 'What do I do now?' "

∎ A growing number of ob-gyns, particularly those in Lyme-endemic areas of California, Wisconsin, Connecticut, New York, and New Jersey, are treating patients prophylactically during the first trimester of pregnancy if they are bitten by ticks or present Lyme symptoms. Dr. Peter Bippart, who is a member of an ob-gyn group in Morristown, New Jersey, sees a significant number of women who have Lyme disease, or are in real danger of contracting it due to tick bites that they have reported.

"In our practice, we will treat a patient with amoxicillin for about three weeks, especially during the first trimester. It is just not worth the risk to ignore it," says Dr. Bippart. "Especially when you consider that the antibiotic treatment is so benign."

SEEKING HELP AND COPING

Although medical viewpoints like Bippart's are slowly spreading, the norm is unfortunately more like the treatment given Diane, particularly in those areas where a massive denial of Lyme disease is prevalent.

If you are pregnant and have been bitten by a tick in an endemic area, are displaying symptoms consistent with Lyme disease, or have been diagnosed with Lyme in the past:

1. Don't accept ignorance or denial from your doctor. During pregnancy, time is of the essence in getting antibiotic treatment to protect your baby if you have, or have been exposed to, Lyme disease. It is important to treat tick bites in endemic areas prophylactically; the comparative risk is minimal.

2. If your doctor refuses to consider Lyme disease, seek help from your local Lyme support group (see appendix A).

3. Don't doubt yourself. If this is a first pregnancy, you may be unaware of the aches and pains that pregnancy causes. If, however, you are not improving or if your symptoms are "different" from those of previous pregnancies and it is possible that you were exposed to Lyme, don't feel "dumb" going back to your doctor and reporting your symptoms.

4. After the birth, be vigilant in your observations regarding the health of your baby. Even though a baby born to a Lyme mother may appear to be healthy at the moment of birth, it is still possible that transplacental Lyme symptoms can crop up months later. There is no need to be paranoid and neurotic about this; just be observant and consider the possibility if chronic illness becomes a way of life for your infant.

5. Breast feeding is also not recommended if you have had

Lyme disease during the previous year since Lyme spirochetes have been isolated from breast milk.

A pregnant woman worries about a lot of things that will affect her baby's health—and rightly so. It is important that doctors realize that, far from being hysterical, most women today are somewhat knowledgeable about their bodies and various health and environmental threats. Complaints of diffuse and migratory symptoms during pregnancy should be treated with respect, not simply dismissed as "pregnant women's blues," curable through Lamaze breathing. Pregnant women must expect and demand this respect and treatment—and seek additional help when they don't receive them.

■ Pregnant women and teens are not the only groups of people who face prejudice or special circumstances surrounding the diagnosis and treatment of Lyme. Senior citizens—however that age is defined—also find that they are lumped into a group with an expected pattern of illness or behavior.

10.
The Elders

If few studies have been done on pregnant women as regards Lyme disease, even less attention has been directed toward the older population. Yet, like the teenager and the pregnant woman, the senior citizen offers a challenge to the diagnosis and treatment of Lyme since more obvious health issues can get in the way.

■ When sixty-four-year-old Tony returned home from a driving vacation through Florida with his wife, he began falling apart. First, he began to forget things—where he was going, what he was doing, the names of friends and relatives. His joints ached so badly that he lost the ability to walk and even to feed himself. Dizzy and confused, he retreated from speaking with people.

When medical help was sought, Tony was quickly diagnosed as having Alzheimer's disease. Three months after he returned from his active trip to Florida, Tony was admitted to a nursing home, incontinent, disoriented, and strapped to a chair to prevent him from falling out.

His distressed daughter, remembering something she had read about Lyme disease, contacted Dr. Derrick DeSilva and asked for an evaluation. After taking a thorough history from family members, reviewing Tony's medical deterioration, and performing an examination and ordering supportive tests, a diagnosis of Lyme disease was made. Tony was put on intravenous antibiotics.

Six weeks later, Tony was once again able to move under his own power, control his bodily functions, and return to his normal life at home, while continuing antibiotic treatment.

■ A case like Tony's dramatically demonstrates how a "catch-all" diagnosis like Alzheimer's can misdirect a doctor's attention from important diagnostic issues when dealing with the older patient. Older citizens get aches and pains; they sometimes suffer a form of dementia. In the not-too-distant past, "Oh, he's just senile" would cover all the bases, including those that caused a personality change as well. It was easy to write off senior citizens because, after all, they were expected to be sickly and would probably die soon anyway.

Today, when modern medicine has allowed us to live longer and octogenarians are the fastest growing age group, even the term "elderly" or "senior citizen" causes confusion. Does one recognize a fifty-five-year-old as a senior citizen, as does the American Association of Retired Persons (AARP)? Or do we address the sixty-five-year-old, who is finally eligible for Medicare, as "senior citizen"? At what point do doctors expect people to begin falling apart?

A CHALLENGING DIAGNOSIS

With Lyme disease, these issues can be very real obstacles to diagnosis. So can the fact that, frequently, older citizens with Lyme may have symptoms masked by other ills such as diabetes, arthritis, ALS, hypertension, heart problems, and some form of dementia. Add to that a prevailing prejudice against the credibility of an older person's memory, and once again we have a situation where a patient must fight to be believed prior to even establishing the illness—and another situation in which an aggressive and caring advocate becomes the patient's best tool for getting proper medical care.

Dr. James Katzel is one who knows. Practicing family medicine in Ukiah, California, which sits at the tip of the Mendocino National Forest and is not far from the famous redwoods, this energetic clinician, who writes a regular Lyme column for a national publication and hosts a weekly radio show, is a throwback to the "good old days." Although only in his forties, Katzel is a firm believer in the necessity of making house calls, particularly when dealing with the more elderly population. He views it as not just a courtesy but as necessary to good medical care.

"House calls are an art form that's coming back into family practice, particularly when dealing with the older segment of the population. Not only do they respond better to the one-on-one treatment, they view it as respectful, and just as importantly, it gives the doctor an opportunity to see how the patient lives, if they have enough to eat, and what other medications they might be taking," says Katzel, who writes a monthly column for the Lyme publication *the ticked-off tract*.

"Having made it to eighty years old, some of these people have a lot of health baggage by the time they come to see you, and the average number of medications they may be taking is three." This has an impact on a diagnosis of Lyme because other antibiotics may cause a false negative test, and other illnesses can cross-react to cause a false positive. For these reasons, the clinical diagnosis leans heavily, once again, on the patient's history.

"History taking is the most important tool a doctor can use at any time, but even more so with an older patient," says Katzel. "But since they may not be able to give it themselves, it is the doctor's responsibility to talk to the children, relatives, even neighbors if necessary, to get an accurate work, vacation, and leisure time history. We also have to look and evaluate whether the symptoms are part of an acute illness or chronic illness, and if the patient is suffering from delirium, whether this is acute as well."

Those patients who are in nursing homes with diagnoses of dementia should be tested for Lyme disease. There is a difference between acute delirium brought about because of Lyme and degenerating dementia caused by other illnesses. The type of dementia caused by Lyme is reversible if it is caught and treated early on in the disease.

Since the older patient will be operating at a disadvantage, both because of the presentations of the illness and possibly because of age, it is very important that a family member or close friend enter into the therapeutic alliance with the doctor to assist in the history taking, asking pertinent questions and assisting the patient in following through on the doctor's recommendations.

Again, as with all other Lyme sufferers, do not accept ignorance or prejudice from your doctor. If you suggest Lyme and the physician refuses to consider it at all or to test for it, then a reevaluation of the doctor-patient relationship may be in order. Be aware that a major consideration in treating older patients is health coverage, whether the patient is with a commercial company or is on Medicare. The ability to pay for treatment once a diagnosis is made influences both the doctor and the senior citizen in accepting a diagnosis of Lyme.

"I DON'T HAVE LYME; I'M CRAZY!"

When Betty decided to retire to one of the great sprawling suburbs of Houston, within an easy drive of the Gulf of Mexico, she thought the golden time of life had finally arrived. Widowed for nearly ten years, the lively sixty-three-year-old had a modest

fixed income, played tennis and golf regularly, traveled, and
loved to sail with friends. In fact, it was sailing that brought her
and her new husband together. Not only did they enjoy the
rigors of hitting the open seas, they equally enjoyed hiking and
camping the rugged hills in the western part of the state. It was
on such a camping trip that Betty feels she must have been bitten
by the infected tick.

"I never saw a rash, but then, I'm outside so much that I'm
pretty tan most of the time. I know, I know, it's not good for
the skin, but there you have it. I never noticed a tick bite. I wish
I had," she says. "It would have made everything a whole lot
easier."

Betty's symptoms began with a flu in September that left her
weak, lethargic, and arthritic. She made the rounds of specialists,
who each began by telling her that a woman of her age had to
expect these kinds of aches and pains, especially when doing
"activities best left for the younger set." She began having problems with her hearing—it would come and go in one ear, alter-
nating with a high-pitched squeal that would last only seconds
yet leave her shaken.

Within weeks, her vision had deteriorated in her left eye,
she could not move without intense pain, she was so dizzy she
could not walk across a room, and she could barely lift her left
arm. She again went through a battery of tests, which came up
negative, and received the doctor's recommendation that she see
a psychiatrist.

By that time Betty's personality had also undergone a
change, and her husband thought a psychiatrist would not be a
bad idea. From the outgoing, energetic, upbeat, and organized
woman he had married, Betty had turned into a depressed, with-
drawn woman whose mood swings ran the gamut from intense
anger to a nearly catatonic state. What she didn't tell her husband
was that she kept getting lost, forgot what she was going to say,
and felt she was going crazy fast. On top of everything else, she

developed bronchitis and her doctor put her on erythromycin, since she's allergic to penicillin. When she woke up one morning to find that her legs did not have the strength to hold her up, she was terrified.

Another round of doctor visits resulted in a diagnosis of acute Alzheimer's. The recommendation was either full-time nursing at home or admittance to a long-term-care facility. It had been five months since her camping trip.

Betty's sister in Southern California badgered Betty's husband into asking for, and then demanding, a Lyme test. Betty tested negative, but her sister wasn't satisfied with the test in view of the antibiotic Betty had been taking for the bronchitis. A few weeks later, they requested a Western Blot that gave a faintly positive reading. Betty was put on an intravenous drug for the four weeks covered by her insurance plan. It was the beginning of a miraculous recovery.

"I actually began to get back to normal," she says. "I was still fatigued and still in a wheelchair, but my muscles began to work again, and I felt I was more in control of my emotions. Just as I was beginning to think I was on my way back to normal, we were told that my insurance coverage had hit its limit on all my tests and expensive treatments. I couldn't believe what I was hearing!"

We will get into the inequities and misguided protocols of insurance companies in chapter 14, but suffice it to say here that Betty had a battle on her hands. The only way to continue treatment, she was told, was for her doctor to diagnose something like a form of mental illness with complications so her office visits, counseling, and therapy could continue. She got back in touch with her sister, who put her in contact with a new doctor. After reviewing her case, this doctor agreed with the Lyme diagnosis and felt longer term treatment was indicated. He agreed to help her get the needed coverage.

Today Betty wears stronger glasses, still has aching joints

on rainy days, and still wakes up in the morning in a "Lyme fog," but she is off antibiotics and walks regularly to get her strength and muscle tone back. And all this was made possible by declaring that she was "crazy," rather than sick with Lyme in a wheelchair, so her medical coverage could be continued.

OTHER TREATMENT CONSIDERATIONS

The cost of treatment is very much on the minds of older patients when they seek the help of a doctor. Particularly if they are on fixed incomes, the doctor's recommendations are measured against the backdrop of mortgage or rent payments, utility bills, and food bills.

"Some patients, if they have to use their money to buy medicine, won't eat well," says Dr. Katzel, "and how are you supposed to get someone well when they aren't eating? This is something the doctor has to be sensitive to.

"Then there is also the issue of compliance. There are two types of older patients—the ones who are obsessively compliant and will do everything the doctor says to the tiniest detail, and those who have no trust in the medical system and won't follow directions at all. This is where the home visits become very useful."

In addition, the treatment of an older patient with Lyme must take into consideration how well the elder's liver is functioning and how well the kidneys are clearing the prescribed medication if the drug of choice is one that settles there. This will be determined through the doctor's history taking, physical examination, and supportive tests.

As we hurtle into the twenty-first century, our definition of "elderly" as well as our concepts regarding the aging process are undergoing dramatic changes. Doctors cannot afford to overlook a possible diagnosis of Lyme simply because the patient falls into a convenient age bracket. The advocate, the therapeutic alliance, and—in the case of the elders, if Dr. Katzel has his way—the home visit will help to assure an accurate diagnosis of Lyme in the senior population, despite the challenges specific to this age group.

11.
Lyme Disease in Animals

What do a cat, a camel, and a giraffe have in common?

Not only are they the only four-legged animals that move legs on the opposite sides of the body at the same time, but despite their diverse geographical habitats they can all get Lyme disease. So can dogs, cattle, horses, rabbits, and many other animals. From Africa to Australia, from Europe to the United States, Lyme disease is hitting the animal population just as surely as the human.

Dr. Dorothy Feir, entymologist and professor of biology at Saint Louis University, points to Lyme disease as the cause of blindness in kangaroos at the Saint Louis Zoo. Cultures taken from the kidneys of the sick animals revealed the presence of the *Borrelia burgdorferi*. In Wisconsin, California, Connecticut, and Missouri, researchers and veterinarians are studying the transmission of Lyme disease among dairy and beef cattle, and even representatives from the Frank Perdue Company, in Salisbury, Maryland, are intensely vigilant in protecting the poultry industry from tick attack. Lyme disease is also on the minds of thousands of horse breeders across the country, because the chronic infection of one horse may result in the loss of hundreds of thousands of dollars.

While comparatively few people are concerned with Lyme in camels, millions are concerned about "man's best friend" because dogs are the prime animal victims of this disease worldwide. It should come as no surprise, since running through tall grass and wooded areas, rolling in fields, and crashing through underbrush rich with ticks is second nature to canines. This can throw their owners into a mass of confusion regarding diagnosis and treatment.

The spread of Lyme in animals parallels the spread to humans in endemic areas, since they are exposed to the same migratory birds and increasingly warmer climates due to the general global warming. In addition, they spend more time out of doors than most humans.

Like their human counterparts, animals generally get Lyme through the bite of an infected tick. As with humans, the diagnosis of Lyme must be a clinical one, as the same weaknesses in testing for antibodies apply. And like humans, these animals can quickly pass from early-stage to late-stage Lyme through a delay in diagnosis, which can render them chronically lame and arthritic.

Unlike most humans, however, animals may contract Lyme from the urine spray of other infected animals, do not usually display an EM rash, and respond to treatment more quickly and with fewer complications.

There are many questions surrounding animals—particularly house pets—and Lyme. The most common include: "Can humans get Lyme from their pets?" "What are the symptoms of Lyme in animals?" and "How can we prevent our pets from contracting Lyme disease?"

DOGS AND CATS AND LYME

Isabelle thought her vet was kidding when he said that all three of her beagles had Lyme disease. Sure they had slowed down (one didn't want to leave its stuffed circular bed), and they didn't

seem to be eating properly, but she attributed that to the fact
that they seemed to eat less in the fall.

But her dogs were prime candidates for the disease since
they lived in an open field area bordered by woods, spent most
of their time out-of-doors, and generally did not require daily
brushing, which might have revealed either the ticks or the rash.

Dr. Barry Lissman, chairman of the Committee on Public
Health and Regulatory Medicine for the New York State Veterinary Medical Society, was the first individual to discover and
report clinical findings on both Rocky Mountain spotted fever
and Lyme disease in dogs. Evaluating clinical findings of Lyme
since 1983, Dr. Lissman won the Award for Outstanding Service
to Veterinary Medicine in 1992 for his original work with Lyme
disease. He feels that anyone living in Lyme-endemic areas should
have their pets tested for Lyme, but they need to be aware that
many animals can test positive yet not show any signs of Lyme.

Says Lissman, "Some animals may have, at some point,
developed a resistance to the disease. The organism may have
been lying dormant in the animal's body or the particular animal
may have better immunity to the organism. Also, the number
and kinds of ticks with which the animal has come in contact
may play an important role in whether or not the animal will
get the disease. Conversely, an animal may test negative and still
have Lyme disease. A history of tick infestation or visits to
endemic areas would be useful in a clinical diagnosis."

While cats can, and do, get Lyme disease, the incidence is
much lower than for dogs. This is partially because they are
primarily indoor animals, and they are better groomers than
dogs, with their rough tongues acting as efficient "brooms" to
rid themselves of ticks. If cats are bitten by ticks, the insects are
more readily seen on the heads and even around the eye areas.

Just as in humans, Lyme disease can affect an animal's
heart, eyes, nervous system, and kidneys. Humans may discuss

"symptoms" of Lyme disease, but since animals can't speak, veterinarians prefer to refer to the "signs" of Lyme. In house pets, these include:

- Arthritis (lameness)
- Lethargy
- Sudden onset of severe pain
- Fever
- Loss of appetite
- Depression
- Other temperament and personality changes

Your veterinarian should be consulted as soon as you observe any of these changes in your pet so he can test for Lyme and rule out other diseases. Both dogs and cats respond quickly to an antibiotic regimen of three to four weeks if the disease is caught in the early stages. But the key to Lyme disease in house pets, as in humans, is prevention.

"Pets and humans should be checked for ticks once or twice a day and more thoroughly after a walk or run outdoors," says Dr. Lissman. "Outdoor areas should be treated periodically with an insecticide approved for use in kennels and/or outdoors. Tall grass, weeds, and brush in the area should be cut, and insecticide powders may help control ticks as will some of the newer permethrin dips and sprays for dogs."

For both small dogs and cats, tick and flea collars recommended by your veterinarian are a good first step in protection. If you should see a tick on Rover or Fluffy, remove it with needle-nose tweezers—not your fingers, nail polish, or a match. As with any tick bite, care should be taken in removing the tick so as not to inadvertently squeeze the "poison" into the animal's system. The tick can then be saved for future identification by placing it in a small, closed container with a blade of grass and/or a piece of damp cotton.

The Fort Dodge Laboratories in Iowa has developed a vaccine that is only designated for dogs at this time. It is given as a series of two injections, three weeks apart, and must be boosted annually.

People cannot catch Lyme disease from their pets, and experts say it is unlikely that a tick that has attached itself to a pet will then "hop off" onto a human. Pet owners just need to be aware that their pets *can* bring ticks into the house, so a thorough daily examination would be in everyone's best interests.

LYME IN CATTLE

Despite the fact that Lyme disease is generally transmitted by a tick bite, there has been some concern that dairy workers could contract Lyme disease from the urine splash of infected cows. Indeed, this appears to be one method of transmission among herds of cattle, according to studies under way at both the University of Connecticut and the University of Wisconsin. Far from being a new manifestation, this came to the attention of researchers when massive cattle herd infection in the United Kingdom resulted in large numbers of animals having to be destroyed.

Although it has not yet been definitely proven, researchers say it is very possible and even likely for the *Borrelia* organism to pass from one cow to another through contaminated urine. Dairy cows are commonly housed closely together on concrete flooring, and it is common for them to sniff around each other's vulvas. But beyond this, when a cow urinates, particularly on a concrete floor, the splash can go as far as three feet, surely far enough to reach the cow's neighbor. (While the active particles of *Borrelia* are present in the urine, once the urine has dried the organism is dead.)

By extension, this theory of infection would support Dr.

Willy Burgdorfer's contention that he contracted Lyme disease from the urine of infected rabbits while he was performing research into Rocky Mountain spotted fever.

Another concern regarding Lyme disease and cattle is whether the organism can be passed to humans via cows' milk or, in the case of beef cattle, through infected meat. Researchers say that, at this time, there is no evidence to suggest that the spirochetes can survive the pasteurization process or any type of cooking process, because heat destroys these organisms as it does other bacteria.

HORSES

Whether a horse costs $4,000 or $400,000, unrecognized and/or untreated Lyme disease can result not only in chronic physical pain for the animal but in emotional devastation and financial burdens for the owner.

Like humans and small pets, horses display a variety of symptoms that may signal Lyme disease and should send up a red flag to call the veterinarian. These include:

- Lameness
- Swelling, pain, or stiffness in the joints of the legs
- Uncoordination
- Fatigue
- Skin hypersensitivity resulting in refusal to be saddled
- Weight loss
- Behavior/attitude changes (i.e., lethargy, aggression, diminished ambition/performance—sometimes referred to as "being a little off")
- Nerve tremors
- Fetal resorptions/abortions
- Nephritis (inflammation of the kidneys)
- Foundering due to laminitis (inflammation of the hoof)

Again, as with humans and other animals, the diagnosis of Lyme disease must be a clinical one, particularly if the blood tests show up negative.

Dr. Jonathan Palmer, an equine specialist at the University of Pennsylvania, says that the important guidepost for diagnosing Lyme in horses is observance of the physical signs of the disease. "It is possible for a horse to be infected by a tick bite and have a negative test result because the animal has not accumulated antibodies yet. It is also possible for a horse to have a positive antibody titer test and be able to fight off the organism without getting the disease. Up to sixty percent of horses will have antibody titers if they live in a Lyme-endemic area, but very few of these will have Lyme disease."

Dr. Palmer says that the industry is looking to depend on the developing reliability of the PCR testing techniques for establishing whether a horse actually has Lyme or not. Until then, a local history of tick infestation, signs of illness, and response to antibiotics remain the diagnostic guidelines.

In treating equine Lyme, veterinarians must also consider the types of antibiotics used, as some common ones can cause undesirable side effects. For example, Tribrissen (a sulfa drug) is not always effective, and doxycycline, which is used in both humans and canines, can produce fatal arrhythmia (abnormal heartbeats) in horses.

■ Currently, there is no vaccine available for animals other than dogs, but the Fort Dodge Laboratories in Iowa does have a multianimal vaccine going through clinical trials. This could be available during the next few years if trials are successful.

III.

GETTING
TREATMENT
AND SUPPORT

■

"Doctors pour drugs of which they know
little, to cure diseases of which they know
less, into human beings of whom they
know nothing."

—Voltaire

12.
Treatment: The Long and Short of It

"I have had two cancers and Lyme disease. With all the pain and suffering that goes along with cancer, I still beat them. I'd trade my Lyme disease for two more cancers any day."

—Cindy M., twenty-eight years old

The definitive treatment for Lyme disease is best expressed by a statement made by Dr. Jorge Benach, professor of pathology specializing in Lyme at the State University of New York, Stony Brook, during a conference in December 1992. He said, "Nothing I say can be taken as gospel truth. It is subject to change, it will very likely change, and will probably be challenged."

In other words, with all that the medical experts and researchers don't know about the Lyme disease spirochete, with all that they do know but are ignoring, and with all that is changing, *there is no definitive and standard treatment protocol for Lyme disease at present*. And that is the crux of the controversy that has polarized doctors, involved insurance companies, and sent ailing patients on lengthy searches for relief. As one patient who has three immediate family members suffering with Lyme said, "What is the problem? Cancer patients don't have to fight for chemotherapy and everyone knows *that* has bad side effects. Why do Lyme patients have to fight for treatment?"

Why, indeed? If we operate from the belief that patients want to get well, and doctors want to heal, it would seem a straightforward matter that doctors would prescribe whatever medication works for as long as it takes to eradicate the symptoms of the disease, thereby assuring that the patient is cured.

As we have already seen, however, nothing is straightforward and simple with Lyme disease, and treatment is no exception.

The controversy arises primarily around the length of time a patient is medicated. Many university-based researchers, who are accustomed to performing controlled studies both in and out of laboratories, maintain that Lyme disease should be "cured" in fourteen to twenty-eight days of antibiotic therapy. It has been proven, however, that antibiotics that seem to work well at eradicating bacteria in the test tube don't perform in the same manner when injected into the human body.

The aggressive clinicians who are swamped with hurting and degenerating Lyme patients maintain that swift and aggressive antibiotic therapy should be continued for as long as the patient has Lyme disease symptoms. This stand is based not only on numerous published research papers detailing the ineffectiveness of short-term therapy for this uniquely potent organism but on the results from literally thousands of Lyme patients who have been treated for varied lengths of time.

Finally, there is a third and growing segment composed of both researchers and clinicians who are weighing all available published data on Lyme with epidemiological evidence and patient histories and are taking a more "middle-of-the-road" approach. They may be aggressively diagnosing Lyme and beginning treatment, yet they are cautious to reevaluate each patient individually as treatment progresses, extending treatment when necessary and providing their patients with adjunctive therapies to boost the body's immune system.

It is these doctors who point to precedents set by the treatment of such things as tuberculosis (another disease with a slow replication rate), which is routinely *initially* treated for six to nine months with multiple antibiotics, and teenage acne, which is routinely treated with antibiotics—uncontroversially—for two years. This has prompted physicians like Derrick DeSilva to say, "If we can treat zits with antibiotics for two years, what is the problem with treating patients ill with Lyme disease for longer than twenty-one days?"

Finally, controversy surrounds the behavior of the organism itself, which has thrown the meaning of the "cure" into contention. It has been documented that the *Borrelia burgdorferi* spirochete can not only change its protein "appearance," once disseminated in the body, but that it can also "hide" from antibiotics within human cells, thus evading eradication by antibiotics. For that reason, this spirochete, like the syphilis spirochete, can go into a dormant period wherein the patient may be free from symptoms, only to relapse when the spirochete flares again.

Although researchers say that a patient is "cured" of Lyme after a specified number of days of treatment, regardless of the symptoms that remain, the majority of clinicians who treat Lyme agree that a patient is not "cured" unless he or she is totally symptom free.

Regardless of a doctor's position on length of therapy, the initial evaluation of the patient's need for antibiotics is based on a classification of symptoms by stages. Depending on the severity of symptoms and the stage of the disease, the doctor will make a recommendation as to whether the patient needs oral antibiotics or intravenous antibiotics, and which type of antibiotics to use.

THE STAGES OF LYME DISEASE

Like most anything else involving Lyme disease, the following chart for gauging the development of the disease is simply a guideline. It is important to remember two things. First, because each person's body is different, one person may pass from the early stage to the late disseminated stage within a few weeks, while another person will take months or even years to progress to that stage.

Second, especially in the early disseminated, late disseminated, and chronic stages, the symptoms do overlap and may vary. One person might have cardiac symptoms associated with early disseminated Lyme, yet be in a chronic stage for everything else.

The chronic stage, defined as having active symptoms for three months or more, includes most of the symptoms from the disseminated stages on a relapsing or chronic basis.

STAGES AND SYMPTOMS OF LYME DISEASE

Early	Disseminated		Chronic
	EARLY	LATE	
EM rash	Headache	Severe headaches/ migraines	Migraines
	Joint pains	Crippling arthritis	Arthritis
	Body aches	Swollen joints	
	Night sweats	Heart blockage	Loss of
	Sensitivity to light, sound, touch	Hypersensitivity to light, sound, touch	libido
	Migratory pains	Crippling	
	Bell's palsy	migratory pains	
	Fatigue	Severe fatigue	Fatigue
	Heart palpitations	Optic neuritis and	
	Swollen glands	increased eye	
	Stiff neck	complications	

Worsening of asthmatic symptoms	Seizures	
	Nosebleeds	Muscle weakness
Disorientation	Memory loss	
Lyme fog	Lyme fog	Lyme fog
Conjunctivitis	Dyslexic reversals	Dyslexia
Sleep disturbances	Sleep disturbances, nightmares	
	Abnormal MRI, CAT scan, EEG, CSF	

COMMONLY USED ANTIBIOTICS

The physician will evaluate a patient's symptoms against the backdrop of the three primary stages before prescribing an antibiotic treatment. Although I will describe the types of antibiotics used, I will not outline prescribed amounts as these not only can change but are up to the individual physician to determine. Suffice it to say that the amounts normally prescribed to attack the Lyme disease spirochete are usually much greater than those normally prescribed for a common bacterial infection.

There are four primary types of antibiotics used to fight Lyme disease, although only one of the classifications was developed with Lyme disease in mind. The others are all general-use, broad-spectrum antibiotics.

The tetracyclines   These include doxycycline and minocycline. While these have been somewhat effective for the early stage of Lyme, many doctors feel that they are ineffective for later stages because they don't penetrate the necessary tissues and systems as effectively as some others.

The tetracyclines are not recommended for pregnant women

or children under the age of twelve, as they can cause the malformation and staining of developing teeth, as well as some blood problems.

The penicillins   Amoxicillin has proven to be a good all-around treatment for early-stage Lyme and, in combination with other antibiotics, for late stages. In addition, it is the only drug of choice at this time for a pregnant woman, as it causes relatively few side effects. It can be administered orally or intravenously.

Sometimes the drug probenecid is prescribed in conjunction with amoxicillin as a booster or facilitator for the antibiotic. It is not recommended for use in children or pregnant women, however, or in anyone with a history of kidney problems.

The macrolides   Erythromycin causes the fewest side effects, but at the same time has proven ineffective as a Lyme antibiotic when used by itself. It may be used in combination with another drug. The advanced azalides, azithromycin (Zithromax) and clarithromycin (Biaxin), have been used for Lyme disease treatment. So far in clinical trials, they seem to be more effective than some other antibiotics in treating later stage Lyme, particularly when neurological problems are involved. Some preliminary work regarding the administering of Zithromax intravenously is being done. At the time of this writing, these two drugs are administered orally.

Because Zithromax and Biaxin are particularly potent, they have an impact on the intestinal tract and must be counterbalanced with nutritional adjunctive therapies (see below) to keep the body on an even keel.

The cephalosporins   The antibiotics from this group are generally second- or third-generation derivatives of other drugs, designed to penetrate a greater number of tissues more effectively.

Ceftin and Suprax are the oral antibiotics; Rocephin and Claforan are the two antibiotics commonly used in IV therapy.

Rocephin has, in some cases, produced gall bladder symptoms, particularly in women. Therefore, Claforan is quickly becoming the drug of choice. As with Zithromax and Biaxin, adjunctive nutritional therapies are recommended to prevent diarrhea and stomach cramps.

There are a couple of other drugs that doctors may prescribe on an individual basis but that are not at this time widely prescribed. These include Primaxin, ciprofloxacin, and Bactrim.

■ If a patient goes to the doctor with an EM rash (early stage), the general consensus is to treat that patient for three to four weeks with amoxicillin. At this point in the course of the disease, aggressive treatment will usually eliminate any further symptoms and dissemination of the disease. The key is to treat early, aggressively, and for a sufficient length of time in order to effect a "cure"—defined as the complete resolution of the disease process or state.

The disseminated stages of Lyme are more difficult to treat because the disease has been carried throughout the patient's body and the spirochete has had an opportunity to establish "hiding" places. If a person has the EM rash and some of the symptoms of early disseminated Lyme, the general choice of treatment would be an oral antibiotic for an initial period of at least four to six weeks. At the end of the initial treatment cycle, the doctor should evaluate the patient for continuing symptoms and signs of infection.

If a doctor sees a patient with late disseminated Lyme, or a large overlap of symptoms, including neurological impairment, he or she will likely put the patient immediately on an IV therapy regimen for an initial phase of four to six weeks, followed by evaluation of the need for continuing antibiotics. At that time, depending upon the patient's symptoms, the doctor may extend IV therapy for another few weeks, or place the patient on oral antibiotics until he or she is symptom free.

During ongoing antibiotic treatment, the doctor should do monthly bloodwork on an "orals" patient, and weekly or bi-monthly bloodwork on an "IV" patient. This will allow the doctor to look for abnormalities in white blood cells as well as monitor the patient's liver functions.

ADJUNCTIVE THERAPIES

One of the concerns patients express is that they have heard that heavy or long-term antibiotic use will destroy the body's immune system and render their bodies defenseless against other infections. This criticism is also leveled by some of the medical critics of longer term antibiotic treatment.

No one can give a guarantee regarding any medical treatment and any medication can cause side effects. Based on long-term antibiotic treatments of such diseases as tuberculosis, urinary tract infections, acne, and children's chronic ear infections, however, there is little reason to suspect that antibiotic treatment of longer than several months' duration will destroy the body or cause subsequent infections to be immune to other antibiotics.

What antibiotics do, however, is diminish the flora in the intestinal tract, which must be replaced to keep the body in balance. For that reason, any Lyme patient who is on a strong antibiotic regimen should add the following to the daily intake:

• Acidophilus—This is the same lactobacillus found in yogurt, but in denser quantities. It replenishes the gastrointestinal flora and prevents the patient from developing yeast infections. While acidophilus is also found in other milk products, as well as in yogurt, the concentration of acidophilus in them is not deemed adequate to offset the reactions caused by the antibiotics; therefore a pill form is commonly recommended.

- Vitamin B complex—helps heal the nervous system.

- A strong multivitamin.

- Vitamin C—if the patient can tolerate it.

- Water—four to six glasses per day are needed to keep the kidneys flushed.

In addition, the Lyme patient should eliminate alcohol intake, as alcohol interferes with the effectiveness of antibiotic action; eliminate sugars as much as possible; and plan on having a rest period each day—prior to exhaustion's setting in.

Other adjunctive therapies, including aerobic exercise, will be discussed in chapter 15.

THE JARISH-HERXHEIMER REACTION

Many Lyme patients who are in the early disseminated stage and beyond will, once placed on antibiotics, experience a period of worsening symptoms—sometimes dramatically—soon after the antibiotic regimen has begun. This is called the Jarish-Herxheimer reaction and is not only to be expected but is actually a good sign that the drug is hitting its target.

Sometimes interpreted by unknowing doctors and patients alike as an allergic reaction to the antibiotic, the Herxheimer (as it is commonly called) occurs when the spirochete, attacked by the drug, gives off toxins and causes the immune system to overreact. It's as though a bomb were dropped on the spirochete, breaking it into ten pieces. Suddenly the body has to fight ten times as hard for a short period of time to eliminate it.

There may be varying degrees of Herxheimer, with additional rashes, headaches, chills, fevers, and lowered blood pressure. *This is a normal and expected reaction.* Do not stop taking your medication should you experience this worsening of symptoms. Do contact your physician, however, and let him or her decide whether you are having a Herxheimer or a real allergic reaction.

Generally, the longer the time between the initial dose of medicine and the Herxheimer, the more disseminated the disease and the longer the treatment may be needed. A Herxheimer reaction can last from two days to two weeks, so a doctor's support is critical.

PULSE THERAPY

Pulse therapy refers to a system whereby a patient gets on a cycle of taking an antibiotic (either orally or intravenously) for several days, then discontinuing for several days. This is called "pulsing."

The theory behind pulse therapy is this: antibiotics kill the spirochete only while it is actively replicating. Not only does the *Borrelia burgdorferi* replicate very slowly, it can become dormant and evade the antibiotics. Thus pulse therapy is based on the idea that the organism will be active and replicate while the patient is off the antibiotics, then can be zapped with a dose when the patient is back on. This is not very different from the pulse therapy used to treat cancer patients going through chemotherapy, and is sometimes used by doctors with patients who have not responded well to other treatments, or who have been on antibiotics for a long time and are still symptomatic.

While it is not recommended or used by all doctors treating Lyme, it has credible advocates. Like any other Lyme treatment, this must be up to the physician and decided on a case-by-case basis. Continuing research should determine the long-term effectiveness of pulse therapy.

PROPHYLACTIC TREATMENT OF LYME

Six-year-old Jenny lives in Saint Paul, Minnesota, and belongs to a family of campers. At least they *were* campers—until Lyme disease brought Jenny's eighteen-year-old brother and her mother to their swollen knees. So when Jenny came home from a friend's house after spending the night and her mother noticed a suspicious dot on the back of her leg during her bath, you can imagine the concern it generated throughout the small family.

Recognizing the tick and removing it carefully, Jenny's mother called the pediatrician and asked that Jenny be put on antibiotics immediately. When the pediatrician assessed the disseminated symptoms suffered by Jenny's mother and brother and acknowledged the fact that they live in a Lyme-endemic area and that Jenny didn't know how long the tick had been attached to her, he agreed.

His decision to put Jenny on amoxicillin for three weeks assured that, should the tick be infected, Jenny would be safe and cured without suffering the same debilitating problems her family members faced. Yet his decision is one that is debated among medical professionals across the country.

At the Fifth International Conference on Lyme Disease, in the spring of 1992, a controlled study was presented showing that even in Lyme-endemic areas there is no benefit to treating a tick bite prophylactically with antibiotics. However, in a paper published by the *New England Journal of Medicine* during the summer of 1992, a study jointly sponsored by the Universities of Colorado and Pennsylvania, Johns Hopkins, and Yale revealed that treating tick bites prophylactically was not only more efficient health-wise but was more cost-effective as well.

This study evaluated three alternatives: (1) empirically treat all patients with two weeks of antibiotics; (2) treat only those in whom the EM rash develops; and (3) treat only those who display an EM rash and have a positive blood test. The results showed that since nearly 50 percent of the people bitten by ticks do not have or remember a rash, by the time other symptoms developed or blood tests were positive, the disease had disseminated throughout their systems and thus presented major treatment and recovery problems. Apart from the common sense of disease prevention, the study also showed that it was more cost-effective all the way around to treat a tick bite for two weeks than to have to institute either oral or intravenous therapy for a longer period of time (not to mention the cost of time lost from work, school, and other activities).

There are still many physicians who do not want to put anyone on an antibiotic unless given irrefutable evidence of infection. There are also those who would probably like to put the entire population of the United States on antibiotics, "just in case." But the majority—particularly those who have treated patients suffering with serious Lyme manifestations—recommend that tick bites in Lyme-endemic areas be treated swiftly and aggressively.

Frankly, *that* is the kind of doctor I would take *my* child to if she were bitten by a tick in this endemic area.

POTENTIALLY DANGEROUS THERAPIES

Any time the public is faced with a disease that causes tremendous distress and is difficult to cure, there exists the possibility of dangerous experimental therapies cropping up as desperate people look for relief. Lyme disease is no exception.

Two experimental therapies that have been tried by patients are malaria therapy and hydrogen peroxide therapy. Those who have tried them say that they were not worth the pain and suffering and did not result in the hoped-for cure.

Malaria therapy is based upon the idea that the spirochete cannot live in a high-temperature setting. Therefore, some patients have traveled to Mexico and other locations to be injected with malaria bacteria, which brings on intense fevers. Not only is the voluntary contracting of a potentially lingering disease such as malaria unwise, but the sanitary conditions under which such treatment is administered, not to mention the purity of the blood and serum being injected, are highly suspect.

Those who have undergone malaria therapy say that in the best of circumstances, relief of symptoms lasted less than two weeks—certainly not enough of a justification for the risks involved.

In hydrogen peroxide therapy, a very diluted hydrogen peroxide solution is injected into the patient in the hope that the chemicals will kill the spirochete. This process is both dangerous and ineffective and should not be attempted.

RELAPSES AND THE DURATION OF TREATMENT

Mark is a thirty-six-year-old architect from San Diego who used to walk around undeveloped properties while planning his shopping center designs. He could have contracted Lyme on any one of his outings or even in his backyard. He was lucky, at first. He tested positive for Lyme disease and his doctor put him on three weeks of antibiotic treatment, during which time he began to feel much better. He could sleep again, the pain in his joints lessened, and his headaches began to decrease in intensity.

At the end of the three weeks, however, his doctor pronounced him cured, despite the fact that Mark still had symptoms. Within the following two weeks his symptoms worsened and then multiplied. When he questioned his doctor, he was told that he had post-Lyme syndrome—that his immune system was still suffering the aftereffects of Lyme and that his symptoms would clear up. When Mark began to suffer tremors and disorientation, and got lost in his own neighborhood, he realized he was not getting better but worse. He spent the next week seeking out another doctor, who began another antibiotic regimen.

At the end of four weeks, he was told he was cured. Afterward, his symptoms again worsened. Mark continued this cycle until he found a doctor who recognized the need for longer and more aggressive therapy. By the time Mark found his current doctor, he was walking with a cane, rarely left his house, and could no longer hold a drafting pencil or sit at his table.

■ In discussing the treatment controversy, it is important for all of us to remember that patients just want to get well. They don't want to get attention or get blitzed—just to be well and normal. Their antibiotic-seeking behavior goes against the normal progression of patient compliance in most other illnesses.

You've probably done it yourself. You know, you're really sick so the doctor gives you ten days' worth of antibiotics. By the third day you're feeling better. By the fifth, maybe you miss a pill because, hey, you're just about well. By day ten—well, we all have antibiotics left over from ten-day regimens we don't bother finishing.

Not so with Lyme disease. Patients who have been diagnosed with Lyme and are painfully symptomatic will put themselves through any torture—including taking all of their medicine—to be well again.

So why won't doctors just give them the medicine? After all, a parent who withholds medicine from a sick child can be charged with child abuse. The only recourse a patient has when confronted by a doctor who bullheadedly declares him or her cured "by the clock," rather than by the eradication of symptoms, is to find another doctor. And he or she should.

The research-oriented conservatives offer as a simple explanation, "We haven't done enough studies to prove that long-term treatment is more effective than two to four weeks'." The interesting fact here is that the standard treatment period of two to four weeks was originally based on comparing the behavior of the Lyme spirochete to that of another spirochetal disease, syphilis. It has since been proven, however, that they don't follow the same initial theory of behavior, but some ideas die hard. This group of doctors acts like a dog who won't relinquish a bone simply because it's his. The difference is that the dog can eventually go off with no ill effects. Doctors who refuse to recognize that Lyme disease can remain active in the system for much longer than the arbitrary two to four weeks are dangerous to their patients.

They are dangerous because they haven't reviewed current literature; because their obstinacy can cause complications and further illness in their patients; and because they influence other, less informed doctors who decide to "go with the flow" rather than read, study, and decide for themselves.

Another influence on the doctors who obstinately maintain that Lyme disease "should be cured in two to four weeks" is that they are often hired by insurance companies that depend on medical professionals not only to advise them on disease treatments but also to justify minimal coverages. This is not to say that all doctors who advocate brief treatment for Lyme are on insurance company payrolls, but some of the major insurance providers in the country today have purposely sought out the most conservative medical element, even in the face of contradictory evidence (more on insurance companies in chapter 14).

To be honest, there have been no curative studies done on Lyme disease at this time. No comparative studies exist on the efficacy of twenty-eight days of treatment versus six months.

There are, however, twenty-four studies showing that four weeks of antibiotic therapy gives incomplete resolution of symptoms, or permits the patient to relapse. These include documentation from reputable and distinguished researchers detailing how active spirochetes have been cultured from the bodies of patients who have completed antibiotic therapies of six months' duration or longer (see the Bibliography).

In fact, Dr. Paul Lavoie, noted rheumatologist and Lyme disease pioneer, said, "I have found evidence for persistent infection in improved patients with ongoing antibiotic therapy of a few years.

"This supports the concept that a bacteriologic cure is not easily achieved by current therapies and that we must not dismiss our patients' complaints following even very prolonged therapy. We must keep an open mind."

There are also ten published articles and at least two general reports showing that longer therapy can give progressive relief, fewer relapses and/or retreatments, and control resurgent symptoms (see the Bibliography).

And in a study completed by the Committee on Infectious Diseases for the American Academy of Pediatrics, Chairman Dr. Stanley A. Plotkin stated: "If all symptoms have resolved, no further therapy is indicated. If symptoms persist, continued therapy is necessary until they have been resolved. Relapses can occur, requiring retreatment with the same or other antibiotics."

In addition, the National Institutes of Health, in a special publication on Lyme disease, concludes: "Later manifestations of Lyme disease are more difficult to treat, sometimes requiring longer and more intensive use of oral antibiotics or intravenous antibiotics, particularly in patients with central nervous system involvement. The efficacy of long courses of antibiotic therapy remains to be demonstrated and needs further study."

Perhaps over the next several years, more doctors will take a more moderate position and gradually a consensus will be achieved.

Dr. Daniel Cameron, an internist and Lyme researcher in Mount Kisco, New York, is accustomed to being on the firing line. He maintains a middle-of-the-road position in terms of treatment, stating that this is where most doctors will be five years down the road anyway. A former academic researcher who headed the National Task Force on Aging, Cameron the clinician is careful to stay aloof from both camps but has a reputation for meticulously challenging researchers at national and international conferences who present papers and theories unsupported by the latest literature. His position represents a growing third "camp" in the Lyme disease medical arena.

"I base treatment on the literature, not the position of my peers. For this reason, I find I am in the middle ground regarding treatment, not diagnosis. I make a diagnosis on clinical grounds. There are many diseases in medicine which we treat even though there may be a low probability that the patient has them, but we do it because, if untreated, they will progress to something much more serious. I feel Lyme disease falls into this category.

"Once the middle ground in Lyme disease is achieved, I think we'll find that doctors will routinely encourage second opinions, and the patient will be better off for it," said Cameron, who is putting together a data base to answer any number of research questions.

The bottom line is that studies will eventually give rise to treatment protocols that will be standardized, with enough flexibility to allow for individual patient response, and the controversy over Lyme treatment will die down. But people who are ill now cannot wait for those studies. Every day that passes for patients with untreated Lyme disease may seal their futures into a pattern of chronic and debilitating illness.

If you have been treated for Lyme for four weeks and still feel ill, you should go back to the doctor and make this clear. Again, do not accept avoidance from your doctor. But remember, too, that your doctor won't know the four-week cure didn't work unless you go back and say so.

13.
Home Care Systems: The Modern House Call

When television's beloved Dr. Marcus Welby routinely stopped by a patient's home to check on her progress and support systems and help solve any myriad of personal problems, grandparents throughout the country nodded, remembering their own kindly doctors from bygone days. During the mid–twentieth century, however, medical care became "hospital centered." Expensive and bulky diagnostic equipment, sterile techniques, and growing populations made it nearly impossible for physicians to routinely visit sick patients at home.

Although physicians who visit homes are still in the minority, a new kind of health professional is once more bringing medical treatment to the home—and the office, and the school—and is sometimes even meeting patients on the road. This is of particular interest to Lyme patients in any stage requiring intravenous therapy since it means that they can continue their lives, for the most part, surrounded by family and engaging in most of the activities they normally enjoy.

Home health care companies have a history stretching back to visiting nurse associations. Modern chronic disease treatments, including those for Lyme, are now often being handled in the home by a specially trained nurse supported by a team of pharmacists, clinicians, and other specialists who work in tandem with the patient's doctor. This nurse will visit the IV patient weekly, change dressings, take a weekly history of progress and/or complaints, assess the supplies, and lend a human touch to the getting-well process. This approach to therapy is often the first time many people have contact with "at home" care.

When Jack, a corporate attorney in Atlanta, was told he had late disseminated Lyme disease and needed to be on IV therapy, he thought his life was over. "I was already trying to hang on while my body was falling apart. When I heard 'IV,' I thought, Okay, now I'm going to be an invalid in the hospital for the next month. It's all over. Boy, what an education I got!" Jack not only had the nurse check his catheter and dressings at the office, he was able to go on business trips and have a nurse from the destination city continue his care.

Emily, a sixty-year-old dairy farmer born and raised in Wisconsin, had slowed some of her activities because of Lyme, but was relieved to find out that she didn't have to stay in the hospital for IV treatments. Twice a day she sat down, hooked up her medication, and read, knitted, or watched television until the forty-five minutes needed for the infusion were up. "Then I hit the barn again."

And Barbara, who despite her Lyme struggled to stay in school, would meet the home care nurse in the school nurse's office. In this way, she was able to keep up with her classes and get the critical supervision she needed.

■ There is a home health care boom going on to the tune of a projected $16 billion by 1997. And although this service is extremely convenient, it places the Lyme patient in an unusual position. After making it through the maze of doctors, tests, increasing symptoms, and finally diagnosis, the patient must then become an employer in a field in which few have expert knowledge.

HOME CARE CONTROVERSIES

Newspaper headlines have appeared in Lyme-endemic areas blasting physicians for referring patients to companies in which they have a financial interest. The implications were that all Lyme doctors who recommend companies are either getting kickbacks or own part of the company.

In other headline stories, home care companies have been exposed as charging inflated prices for medication. Where two grams of Rocephin, prescribed as one gram twice a day, may cost $170 through one company, another might charge up to $450 for the same two grams.

And some insurance companies and HMOs, as well as Medicare, have been reluctant to cover portions of—or any—therapies provided by home health care companies. They have charged that money-hungry doctors refer patients for IV therapy even when they don't need it because the health care companies give the doctors kickbacks for those referrals.

What is a patient to do when confronted with another confusing choice after having IV therapy prescribed? The smart medical consumer will ask questions, and a lot of them, right from the beginning.

TWO TYPES OF IV THERAPY

Depending upon the patient's age and stage of Lyme disease, life-style, and the accessibility of veins, the doctor will recommend that either a "peripheral catheter" or a "central line" be put into the patient's body for administering medication.

Peripheral catheters are usually inserted into a vein in the forearm, although individual circumstances may occasionally dictate another site. This insertion is easily performed in the doctor's office, and the catheter (often called a Pic Line, Stream-line, or Landmark) can remain in the patient's arm, barring complications, for anywhere from two to six weeks before it needs to be removed or replaced. Medication is infused through the vein, either by gravity (the traditional hanging bag) or through one of several "IV push" methods, which can include portable containers or time-release pumps.

A central line catheter is implanted in the chest area by a surgeon, and the medication goes directly into a vein, which transfers it directly into the heart. This central line, usually referred to as an "implanted port," can remain in a patient for months before needing replacement. The site for medication infusion would be in either the upper arm or the chest area, and infusion is accomplished in the same ways described for the peripheral line.

Both types of lines are easily camouflaged by clothing and do not cause discomfort to the patient if inserted properly. One primary restriction is that they should not become wet or be immersed—this means no swimming and that care must be taken when bathing. Following the initial insertion, done either in the doctor's office or in an ambulatory surgery unit, the continuing monitoring and care of the IV line is then referred to a home health care company.

When a physician prescribes IV therapy, he or she may make a recommendation for a preferred home health care company. The hardest thing to remember at this point is that you, as the patient or advocate, have a choice. For many who have searched for a diagnosis, the doctor who finally pinpoints Lyme disease may seem to wear wings and a halo, and they may be earned. But asking the right questions is part of your therapeutic alliance, and a reputable doctor will be straightforward in giving reasons for preferring a company and will encourage you to make some telephone calls before coming to a decision.

AM I COVERED?

Prior to selecting a home health care company, you should begin by contacting your insurance company to find out what it will cover in terms of home care. Since there are some policies that do not cover home care at all, you must first make this determination. If you have established that your company *will* cover some portion of home therapy, the following questions should be asked:

1. What is my deductible for home health care?
2. Is IV therapy covered entirely if taken at home or must I be in the hospital for some portion of it?
3. What percentage of the therapy is paid by the insurance company and what do I have to pay?
4. Is there a maximum benefit for home IV therapy, after which the company will discontinue coverage? What is that amount?
5. Does the company have a "case management" policy once the client has amassed large bills? This may indicate reassessment of the medical situation with the possibility of reduced coverage.
6. What is the name of the person with whom you will be dealing?

Once you have established the insurance company's coverage, the first decision to be made is whether to go with a local, national, or international home health care company.

SELECTING THE COMPANY

When ten-year-old Billy was diagnosed as needing intravenous therapy for disseminated Lyme disease, his mother, Marsha, decided to go with a local company. She knew the director of nursing and, in fact, had worked with her on a fund-raiser at church. Dealing with this company was like having a neighbor watching over her son. This was a relationship that worked well.

∎ Carl needed a company that could accommodate his business travel schedule. As Midwest sales manager for a large pharmaceutical firm, he sought out a home health care company that could continue his IV supervision on the road, if need be. This relationship also worked well.

∎ Carol also traveled, but her business travel as a fashion representative included trips to London, Paris, Rome, and sometimes Hong Kong. In order for her to continue working while on IV therapy, she needed to find a company that could accommodate *her* schedule, since overseas travel was usually a little less flexible than domestic. She, too, found a company that could provide continuity despite her location.

∎ There are thousands of home health care companies—and many more springing up on a monthly basis—so it may seem a daunting task to sift through the names and make a decision as to which one would be right for your particular situation. Your first consideration should be whether to go with a company that is local, one that has offices in other states, or one that can serve you not only locally or nationally but internationally as well. The three that I have chosen to present here have all been in business nearly ten years, or longer, and are fully accredited by both of the major watchdog organizations. There are many equally good companies in various locations throughout the country. The information given here is simply to be used as a guideline in selecting a company.

All things being equal (and we will discuss accreditation, personnel training, and services below), if the Lyme patient is not likely to travel out of state during the treatment, a local company would be ideal.

"One of the major advantages to using a local company is that we have community contact with our patients," said Maggie Davidson, director of Alliance Home Care Company, based in Cedar Knolls, New Jersey. It presently services a six-county area. "I see my patients in the grocery store, on the Little League teams, and around town shopping. The close contact emphasizes the importance of professionalism on our part, and kindness and caring, because these are literally our neighbors. And if something goes wrong with an IV, or someone is worried about their care, we are there in minutes to help him or her through the problem."

U.S. Home Care is a company that began on a local basis in the late 1970s but decided to spread into the national arena. Based in Hartsdale, New York, it began its expansion primarily to satisfy the needs of working patients, according to Michele Rosenblum, vice president of patient services. "We are talking about a population that wants to continue to work, despite the need for therapy. They want to continue a normal life, and we believe that we are in a position to remantle the dismantled patient in this age of specialties. People expect respect in their own homes, and want to be treated like human beings whether they are sick and on the road or at home."

Caremark, also in business since the late seventies, has more than eighty sites throughout the continental United States, and facilities in many of the major world capitals. "At this point, no place is inaccessible to us," said Diana Florio, payor relations manager. Although Caremark's corporate headquarters are in Chicago, clients throughout the country who find that business or vacations take them on the road or across any of the oceans can continue their IV treatments, with their medications cleared through customs and their documentation established.

Once you have chosen the type of company, you should check the organization's accreditation. As of this writing, the accreditations needed vary from state to state. One standard of excellence, however, is whether the home health care company is Joint Commission Accredited, or Home Caring Council Accredited. These are voluntary certifications that require stringent guidelines for training, service, and quality control.

After having ascertained the company accreditation, you should then begin with the critical questions.

ASKING THE RIGHT QUESTIONS

Reputable home health care companies should be judged in three basic areas: patient services, personnel, and quality control. These three areas can be further broken down. The following guidelines can be used when shopping for a company.

■ Patient Services

1. Do you have a twenty-four-hour-a-day emergency number? What is your response time?

Whether you choose a local, national, or international company, home health care is all about providing local service on demand. The larger companies should have a local office from which they dispense medications and personnel. Emergencies and concerns arise at all hours of the day and night, and a patient should be able to call the company and have a nurse visit at three

A.M. if necessary—and do so cheerfully and competently. Most reputable companies will have someone at your front door within fifteen minutes to half an hour.

2. What materials do you provide for patient education?

After the first dose of medication, which should be given in the doctor's office, and the first instruction on how to administer the medication yourself, the company should provide the patient and advocate with educational materials. This should not only include a step-by-step chart of how to administer the medication, but a "what if" list of possible concerns, signs of problems, and possible solutions, including calling the nurse. Some companies, like U.S. Home Care, provide their Lyme patients with professionally produced videos, while others provide booklets, charts, and notebooks. "It's important that companies provide written instructions to their patients because we are dealing with people who are sick and anxious; they won't always be operating at their normal capacity," said Diana Florio.

3. Do you encourage patient participation?

This covers everything from patients feeling at ease in asking questions outside the normally assigned appointment to reassuring patients as to where their responsibilities lie. This may be particularly important when a child needs infusion therapy.

"Sometimes parents need the reassurance that we [professionals] are responsible for doing the sticking and inserting," said Davidson. "If a child is old enough to infuse their own medication, we certainly work with them and encourage this kind of responsibility. Sometimes, when you have multiple family members down with Lyme, the medication schedules can get a little confusing, particularly if people are suffering from short-term memory loss. We work with them on setting up the sched-

ules, lists, and checking the medications off daily, to make sure
everyone has theirs."

4. Are your charges line charges or bundled?

Upon being interviewed, some companies may tell you that
each dose of Claforan will cost you $200. What you need to find
out is whether this figure applies just to the medication (a line
charge), with separate charges for the nurse visit, the equipment,
and twenty-four-hour emergency service, or whether it includes
all those services as well as the medication (a bundled charge).
Make sure you are comparing apples and apples when shopping
for a company.

5. Will IV therapy be provided at various sites at the patient's convenience?

One day, the patient may need to be met at work in a
particular time slot, or at school, rather than at the "normal"
home location. Make sure your company has this flexibility.

6. What kind of support services are available?

Well-established and reputable companies will either offer,
or have access to, a variety of services such as nutritional counseling, research data on Lyme disease, insurance company liaisons,
and personal assistance in such areas as grocery shopping, bill
paying, and transportation. Of particular importance is the company's help in dealing with insurance companies, as its personnel
will likely have more experience in dealing with therapy reim-
bursements than the clients.

"Insurance companies are going more into managed care as
a type of service, and may have to precertify your Lyme disease
and then follow it carefully," said Florio. "The therapies provided by a home care company are less expensive than if a patient
were confined to a hospital, but they aren't cheap, so working
with the insurance company for the patient's benefit is crucial."

■Personnel

7. Do you provide a uniform standard of procedures for your nurses?

There are many skilled and experienced nurses from many fine institutions that teach IV procedures in very different fashions. One of the aspects of therapy you are "buying" from a home health care company is consistency in quality care. The company should provide an orientation and standardized process not only for its nurses but also for those who answer the telephone, deliver the medications, and assist patients in any of the supportive services.

8. Do you have a specially trained pediatric IV nurse available?

This should be insisted upon when the patient is a child, said Davidson. "Not all nurses who have been trained on IV therapy have experience dealing with children, and this is critical. The emotional overlay in the family is different when it is the child on IV therapy. The technical aspect of working with smaller veins is more challenging, and adolescents and teens, in particular, are very body-conscious. You need a nurse who is sympathetic, experienced, and skilled in dealing with all these issues. Insist upon it; it's part of what you are paying for."

9. What type of ongoing training or assessment do you provide your staff?

Home care is personal care, and *everyone* who comes in contact with the patient—from the person answering the telephone to the person who delivers the weekly supply of medication—should be accessible, helpful, and kind. One can get a sense of the company's standards simply by calling and asking a few questions. The more reputable companies will invite you in for a tour; your questions will be answered patiently and completely. You should never feel as though you are imposing on them. Remember, *you* are the boss who is prospectively hiring *them*, and you should be treated as such.

Many times, particularly with older patients who are reluctant to ask questions or complain to a nurse, the delivery person becomes the front-line representative for the company. There should be a system of feedback so that a patient's concerns can be reported to the case nurse or supervisor.

10. Can we change nurses if a problem occurs?

Not every nurse-and-patient combination is made in personality heaven. Despite a high competency level, the chemistry may just be off. Or the patient may have a legitimate concern about the nurse's skill. In both of these situations, the patient should have the right to change nurses without any anxiety of reprisals or an implication of "snitching." After all, you would have few reservations over complaining about service at a restaurant. Why should you show your health any less respect?

11. Do you have pharmacists on staff? Where? May I speak with them about my medication?

Again, whether a company is local, international, or in between, home health care is a local service and a patient has a right to speak with the pharmacist in charge. Beware the companies that have only technicians, or a consulting pharmacist. This is your life you are putting in their hands, and you want assurance that your medications are correct, fresh, and given personal attention.

12. Where is the closest office to me?

"Home health care is a local market; procedures that may work in New York may not satisfy a patient in rural Georgia or Florida," said Rosenblum. Nurses, drivers, and pharmacists should be local and "on call," with backup available twenty-four hours a day.

13. Do you pay physicians for referrals?

While this varies from state to state, it is generally a law that any physician who has a financial interest in a health care company to which he is referring patients have a public announcement card placed in a very visible location in the office. By the same token, it is "illegal and inappropriate to pay physicians for referrals," said Florio. "The question then arises, 'Is the physician earning so much with a home care company that he has an incentive to send patients into therapy even when it's not necessary?' Patients should ask about a doctor's financial interest in the company before making decisions about it."

■ Quality Control

14. How large a supply of equipment is delivered at a time? If we run out of something, can it be replaced?

Reputable companies will not deliver more than a week's worth of equipment for IV therapy (bandages, tape, syringes, saline, heparin, etc.) at a time. In addition, each patient must be supplied with an anaphylaxis kit in case of allergic reaction.

The visiting nurse should do an equipment assessment at each visit, with a follow-up telephone call from the company. A patient shouldn't have to run out to the drugstore to pick up rolls of tape. The thing to remember is that once the equipment has been delivered to you, it cannot be returned and recycled. (At least it should not be!) Therefore, you want enough to make it through the week, but not so much that you are wasting money on excess supplies.

15. How do you track a patient's progress?

A number of companies use the "one chart" system, whereby each person has a chart that contains contributions from not only the case nurse but the physician, pharmacist, delivery person, and anyone taking telephone calls from the patient. In this way, each patient's information is organized and complete. Other companies have giant display boards at the office, with each patient's information listed on a weekly basis. It is important for you, the medical consumer, to know that your therapy is part of a coordinated effort.

16. How often does the company have contact with my doctor?

Again, this goes back to coordinated care and open communication. Home health care is a team effort to get the patient well, and the physician and home health care professionals must keep each other apprised of any changes in the patient's condition. An attentive home care nurse will inform the patient's doctor of any changes on a routine basis.

17. Does the agency write a personalized care plan for each patient?

This may be a foregone conclusion if the home care company is accredited by the two large voluntary commissions, but it's a good question to ask nonetheless.

■ Finally, as with anything else, the best recommendation is word of mouth from those who have been through the same experience. If you are confused over home health care companies, begin by asking your physician or by contacting members of your local Lyme support group to find out which companies might successfully offer those services that satisfy your individual needs.

14.
What's Insurance For?

People in Donna's old neighborhood called her family "the Lymies," but Donna, facing financial devastation, isn't laughing. The forty-four-year-old nurse and her three daughters are all victims of Lyme disease. Tina, fifteen, and Ceil, thirteen, have been on intravenous treatment intermittently for two years. Tina, who suffers from severe eye pain and loss of peripheral vision and has difficulty concentrating, is unable to attend school regularly and studies at home with a tutor's help.

Ceil, who is currently on intravenous treatment, goes to school part-time. She, too, has headaches, joint pain, neurologic impairment, dizziness, and fatigue.

Karen, the eight-year-old, displayed few symptoms until she began having episodes of tremors. Then the joint pain, stomach cramps, headaches, and heart palpitations kicked in.

In the spring of 1992, Prudential Insurance informed Donna that she and her daughters should be well, that further treatment was deemed not medically reasonable by the company, and that further medications and services for Lyme disease would not be covered.

Donna, a single parent, is particularly upset because she had been buying medical supplies directly from the hospital and administering the medication herself, rather than paying a home health care company. Despite the savings, she has been forced to sell her home and borrow from relatives in order to meet the cost of medical treatment. Not only is she upset, she is angry. "I am outraged to be told by an insurance company that, according to their textbooks, we are supposed to be well, so they aren't paying for our medical treatment. Is this why I have contributed to their company for all these years? Since when did insurance companies get medical degrees?"

■ By now, it is fairly common knowledge that more than 35 million Americans cannot afford health insurance. For those people, even a simple procedure is costly. But even many of those 177 million Americans who *do* have health insurance are finding that their insurance is anything but a guarantee when it comes to covering the cost of an illness like Lyme disease. More than 39 million people presently enrolled in the once-enticing HMOs find that their coverage does not extend to doctors and treatments for various specified diseases, such as Lyme disease. And by the year 2000, up to 30 percent of all working and retired adults who purchased long-term-care insurance, labeled the fastest growing type of insurance today with more than a million active policies sold, may find themselves "uncared-for" if their health problems are due to Lyme.

Currently, the guidelines of some of the nation's largest carriers will not allow for retreatment or extended treatment of Lyme disease, and the initial treatment period is deemed to be twenty-eight days. This is in spite of documentation from around the country that a significant percentage of patients are outside of the "early treatment" parameters due to late diagnosis and the pathology of the organism itself.

At a March 1992 meeting convened by Congressman Chris Smith of New Jersey, with the heads of two divisions of the National Institutes of Health, the Centers for Disease Control, and Lyme disease patient advocacy groups, a spokesman for NIH said that therapeutic decisions should be based on the clinical response of the patient and the judgment of the doctor. While this sounds theoretically supportive, the harsh realities of insurance coverage have increasingly put Lyme patients in the no-win situation whereby one company declares them well and therefore ineligible for continued coverage, yet another company labels them as having a preexisting condition if they attempt to apply for new insurance.

In addition, because states are prohibited from regulating self-insured employers under the Employee Retirement Income and Security Act (ERISA), employees' coverage can be pulled at any time, and smaller insurance companies have the option of canceling policies of the sickest patients in order to save money. This was evident when the state of California gave permission to the Great Republic Insurance Company to cancel fourteen thousand policies overnight, including those of a woman who had just learned she had cancer and a man scheduled for heart surgery.

Many insurance companies, utilizing the medical profession's own competing factions and polarity regarding Lyme disease, maintain that treatment beyond thirty days is experimental and noncurative. Clinicians and patients, pointing to continuing published research discoveries and the individual's own response to therapy, angrily charge that insurance companies are not fulfilling their contractual obligations, are practicing medicine without a license, and are forcing policyholders and their children into chronic ill health and financial ruin when the client finally attempts to collect on paid-up policies.

There are insurance companies with integrity across the country that *are* covering their policyholders who contract Lyme. Unfortunately, these are too few and far between—but they have earned the undying loyalty of their clients. The fear of losing coverage is so great among Lyme patients, however, that in interviewing people across the country, I was repeatedly begged *not* to mention the names of these reputable carriers because their clients are terrified that their companies will join the bandwagon of dumping Lyme patients.

The major insurers have traditionally had the credibility of institutional status and billions of dollars of assets in their arsenal of weapons against a policyholder's claim. Yet thousands of sick "Davids" are developing new weapons and girding themselves to take on these heretofore intimidating "Goliaths." The outcome of this face-off could influence the future of insurance underwriting.

THE INSURANCE EDGE

People buy insurance as protection against and compensation for adversity. The concept, as it originated, seems simple enough. Mr. X pays Company A ten dollars a week for health coverage. When Mr. X gets sick, the company is expected to pay the bills, as set forth in the original agreement. Whether Company A makes or loses money along the way is generally immaterial to Mr. X, as long as he receives what he has paid for when he needs it.

As the theory progressed to industry status and simple policies mutated into a cornucopia of variables, insurance companies, now inflated with investments, landholdings, personnel, and self-importance, began changing the rules of the original game when faced with situations that affected the bottom line. This is all the more upsetting to the American public because it views the insurance industry not merely as a business but as a caretaker of health and welfare. After all, these companies are influencing the course—and sometimes the end—of people's lives.

This pluralistic view finds little sympathy in an industry that avows allegiance first to its shareholders, and second to its policyholders. Representatives complain that the public wants more and unlimited coverage for less money. The public complains that it has paid high premiums for years (health insurance costs comprise more than 20 percent of the Detroit automakers' total wage bill, for example), only to be cut off when needs arise.

Collectively, Blue Cross and Blue Shield companies probably represent the largest health insurance carrier in the country. Approximately half of the Blue Cross claims by Lyme patients applying for extended treatment have been denied. Other giants such as Prudential and Aetna also uphold the "four weeks of therapy is sufficient" treatment for Lyme disease.

During the summer of 1992, an insurance company spokesperson warned in the *Asbury Park Press* (Asbury Park is located in an endemic area) that doctors who "overreport" cases of Lyme disease will be investigated for fraud and abuse, and such reports must be predicated on the CDC's admittedly restrictive criteria for Lyme disease. In response, the CDC has emphasized that its criteria are not to be used by doctors or insurance carriers for defining Lyme disease, but the intimidation tactics employed by the carriers against doctors have already dissuaded many from diagnosing and treating ill patients.

Dr. Stanley Harris trained as a pediatrician and worked his way up through the medical hierarchy, managing eleven acute care hospitals and multiple health centers in the New York City system before finally sliding into the position of associate medical director for Blue Cross, Blue Shield of New Jersey. His state is the third highest in the nation in Lyme disease claims, only slightly behind New York and Connecticut. Despite the fact that he has attended Lyme disease conferences and met with clinicians who treat multitudes of patients, he says that the policy of the company to stick to the thirty-day coverage is based on published literature, admittedly conservative academic experts, and the lack of comparative studies.

"We want every decision to be as accurate and representative of what's going on out in the field as possible, and the way we approach Lyme disease is the same as our approach to other diseases. We are looking for medical evidence which has been put through scientific replication. We know there is a great deal of difference between the individuals who are daily treating and practicing medicine and those affiliated with an academic medical setting. There are few medical therapies out there that don't have some controversy, from asthma to cancer treatments. But not every circumstance involves the patients and their whole families the way Lyme disease has done. We are not telling doctors that they must practice in a certain way; we're just saying that after thirty days, we won't cover the treatment at this time.

"If there are those out there who are finding consistent results in their treatments, I encourage them to put these on paper so they can be replicated."

Harris says that Blue Cross and other insurance companies do tend to turn to academic and medical centers for second opinions and consultations because of their inherent status as teaching centers, but that there is a recognized potential for bias. This kind of issue goes back to the conflict between the two groups of doctors and the lack of comparative treatment studies—all by-products of the "growing pains" of this disease.

Another weapon in the arsenal of insurance company claims offices is the bureaucratic tap dance done on appeals of company policy.

Kevin, his wife, and his daughter all contracted Lyme disease while on a family vacation in the Southwest. Since it affected each differently, taking varied times to disseminate and become debilitating, they were each in varied disseminated late stages before the disease was diagnosed and treatment begun. Four weeks into the treatment, their insurance company discontinued coverage. All three family members began sliding backward when treatment was stopped. Kevin's twelve-year-old daughter began having tremors and heart palpitations, which landed her in the hospital. They began the process of appealing the insurance company decision.

While Kevin filled out the necessary appeal forms and waited, he took out a second mortgage on his house and depleted his savings in an attempt to pay for continued IV therapy. Weeks passed, during which the company said it had misplaced the file, please file again; the caseworker was on vacation; the file had to go to the home office; the file had to go to medical consultants; the caseworker quit and a new caseworker needed time to acclimate; the file was misplaced, would he please file again?

At the end of nine weeks, and still with no response from the insurance company, Kevin had to give up his own treatment so he could continue to pay for his family's. At the end of eleven weeks, his wife gave up her treatment so their daughter could continue to fight Lyme.

Today Kevin is in litigation with his insurer. He is in a wheelchair; his wife uses a cane. Their daughter is off IV therapy and on oral antibiotics but is suffering from depression and guilt, feeling she is to blame for her parents' debilitated condition.

As one West Coast physician, who has counseled numerous patients on fighting for their paid coverage, says, "We send the charts, the charts get lost. We recopy them. The company changes personnel. I would have to stop practicing medicine and just spend my days helping patients fight the insurance companies if they were to be successful. That's what the companies count on; they know we don't have that kind of time and the patients are often too sick to follow through. The vicious circle is that, if they don't follow through, they get even sicker. Either way, the patient loses."

This underscores the need for a patient advocate, as it would become the advocate's responsibility to assist the ill person in petitioning for continued coverage. On a more formal basis,

Lyme patients across the country may have found representation through independent organizations formed to do battle with the insurance industry.

PATIENTS FIND A VOICE

Anne Ebert's battle with Lyme began more than ten years ago when her eighteen-month-old son displayed the classic bull's-eye rash and her doctor told her not to worry because "blonds get all kinds of rashes." Although he was mentally bright, the child's physical development was slow as he grew, and he suffered from continual illnesses. As a Girl Scout leader from 1979 to 1984, Anne pulled deer ticks off all her charges, including her two daughters and her son, who began the cycle of illness. Then a cherished family vacation to Germany's Black Forest brought Lyme disease to the forefront of the Ebert household. Little did Anne know that the tick bites she and her three children got there were to complicate their Lyme disease diagnosis back in the United States.

The Eberts tested positive for Lyme, but Anne's son was the hardest hit. After being treated for twenty-eight days, he got better, but when treatment stopped, he plunged into a deeper illness and paralysis. Treated again, along with his sisters, the boy began to get better once more. Then Anne and her husband were informed that the insurance company would no longer pay for treatment. Three days later, their son collapsed.

"You have to be a fighter," said Anne, who contacted the local television station and told them that a twelve-year-old boy's life was on the line. "And you have to have help because Lyme patients are often not capable of rocking the boat because they are so sick."

Anne's three-year battle for insurance coverage took on formal status in 1992 with the formation of VOICE (Victims of

Insurance Company Exploitation). With experience gained from long-ago civil rights marches, Anne organized VOICE to force insurance companies to live up to their contractual obligations in covering patients. Her fight interested New Jersey State Senator John Bennett, who introduced a bill requiring insurance companies to fulfill their contractual obligations or be banned from doing business in the state.

The attention of insurance companies and patients across the country was fixed on the packed New Jersey Senate hearing chamber in December of 1992, when Bennett addressed insurance representatives, doctors who had closed their practices for the day, and Lyme patients, many of whom leaned on canes or on the walls for support. He stated unequivocally, "When people buy insurance policies, they expect that it will cover them for all disease. I don't think it should be necessary to have families faced with the loss of their homes. The families who need treatment, while waiting for us to decide this bill, will lose their resources paying for medication." At the time of this writing, the New Jersey State Senate had passed the bill and it was scheduled for final presentation to the full assembly. It faces strong opposition from major insurance carriers.

While her difficulties have frustrated Ebert, who herself deals with the effects of relapsing Lyme, they don't dissuade her, as word of Lyme activism has spread. "I learned long ago that working within the system is the most effective method of making changes, and that the system does work but it needs a lot of prodding."

Dr. John Bleiweiss, a Trenton, New Jersey, internist who treats hundreds of Lyme patients, has been prodding newspapers, institutions, and legislators with facts regarding the need for long-term treatment in cases of disseminated Lyme. Armed with both clinical experience and published research, he scoffs at what he terms the "Bermuda Triangle logic" of those companies denying their Lyme patient policyholders treatment coverage.

"In a letter to a patient of mine, an insurance company wrote: 'There seems to be no documentation that the patient did in fact have Lyme disease' and 'there is no documentation of central nervous system Lyme disease.' This patient [who had been diagnosed with Lyme on the recommended clinical basis] had severe cognitive impairment demonstrated on neuropsychiatric examination by an independent clinician," says Bleiweiss. "He also had many of the cognitive problems that can be resolved using prolonged IV and oral antibiotic treatment. The patient, now on pulse therapy, continues to improve." If some parts of the medical community still say this type of successful long-term treatment isn't sufficient "clinical proof," then many other accepted treatments now used successfully aren't justified either. These include the prescribing of Inderal for migraine headaches and nitroglycerin for treating chest pain.

"Insurance company consultants have not been able to prove that twenty-eight days of treatment for Lyme is curative. On the contrary, abbreviated therapy in many patients permits survival of the Lyme disease spirochete and fails to provide enduring symptom relief. This has been established through published research studies over the last year. Often, symptoms return within one to two months after a short course of antibiotics. Dr. Burrascano and others have reported that patients had progressive relief and fewer relapses with longer antibiotic treatment, whether IV or oral. I feel the insurance companies have adopted an inappropriate standard of care which is inconsistent with the available research and patient experience."

The insurance industry's stated policy of not covering treatment beyond thirty days because such treatment is not curative and is "therefore experimental" doesn't hold water when one looks at its coverage of other diseases that—unlike Lyme disease—do not have a definitive cause or endpoint. Illnesses such as fibromyalgia, chronic fatigue syndrome, chronic mono, or even multiple sclerosis have stumped the researchers for years and their sufferers number in the millions. Yet for as long as symptoms are present, treatment is covered.

The bottom-line decision by insurance companies not to cover Lyme patients beyond a limited time is a financial one, until such time as the research overwhelmingly, unequivocally, and consensually dictates certain treatment paths. And even then, says a former insurance claims investigator, many companies will still do everything in their power to cancel their clients' policies.

THE "EVERY CLAIM IS A FRAUD" MENTALITY

David Testone, of Brewster, New York, went to work for Mutual of Omaha after teaching school for ten years. He proved such a capable pupil during his eleven months of training that he was assigned to the company's special section—or the SS, as it was referred to—the function of which, Testone maintains, was primarily to stalk those who filed claims and find evidence to cancel their policies. The prevailing mind-set in much of the health insurance industry is that every claim is fraudulent and should be treated as such.

He worked thirty-five states, along with sixty of the "chosen SS," and was often told, "Handle claim accordingly." "It was our code phrase meaning to do anything and everything it took to pull the policy. The intimidation tactics I used were unbelievable," he says. "I characterize myself as having become crude, cold, and callous. I once took away a policy from an elderly man in a hospital bed in his house. I'm not proud of things like that."

Four years ago Testone reassessed his life and the industry and teamed up with Ron Alford, of Manhattan, a former Prudential employee and author of *Crime of the Century*, an exposé of the insurance industry, to jump the fence and help policyholders fight for their rights. The two have been on numerous television shows, including "Hard Copy," and Testone is vociferous in his condemnation of insurance tactics.

"There is no doubt in my mind that insurance companies are practicing medicine without a license. They don't want to pay claims, period. I had one insurance company guy tell me, 'Look, with AIDS patients, we know there's an endpoint; they'll die. With Lyme disease patients, we could be on the hook forever.' "

Testone says that with some companies, you're damned if you do and damned if you don't—meaning that if you file a Lyme disease claim for treatment at a teaching hospital or center, the claim is flagged because it is assumed the prices are inflated. If the claim is filed for treatment by a clinician, it is discarded if it's not in sync with the recommendations of an academic teaching institution. What to do?

"Lyme disease patients have to get involved politically," says Testone. "They are ten years behind AIDS patients in getting their rights. You can't just have conferences and talk about the problem and not get anything accomplished. You have to put your legislators against the wall and make them accountable. And look at who's funding those legislators' campaigns. If insurance companies are on the list, there's a good reason for that.

"People get intimidated by the insurance companies and walk away. And the insurance companies—the ones that aren't paying—are getting away with murder. Lyme disease is the biggest scam going in the insurance industry now. The medical providers cannot agree amongst themselves on treatment and they are unwittingly doing the dirty work for the companies, which are using those disagreements to not pay, without getting their hands dirty."

Equitable treatment from insurance companies is also the province of Families USA, located in Washington, D.C. Formerly the Villers Foundation, it was founded in 1981 by Philippe Villers and his wife, Kate, to reform the health care system in the United States so that it assures universal access to care. Villers, who fled to the United States when he was five years old to escape Nazi persecution, grew up to become the creator of Computervision, a successful computer company. The foundation is his contribution to his adopted country. It provides grants and advocacy for those seeking redress in the health care arena, and has a membership of 135,000 in the advocacy arm alone. Phyllis Torda, director of health and social policy for the organization, says that they cannot do anything for Lyme patients until complaints are filed with them. When they hear from patients, they will then be able to swing into action.

A WEAKNESS IN MANAGED CARE

By the end of 1991, more than 39 million Americans were enrolled in a health maintenance organization (HMO). This attractive alternative requires only small fees for doctor visits and provides special services not found in traditional insurance plans, like coverage for annual checkups or "well visits." It offers a variety of services for a little bit of money, which sounds like a bargain. And it is, if you don't get something like Lyme disease.

One of the restrictions of an HMO is the limited pool of doctors a patient can visit. Marie's daughter, who was experiencing numbness and tingling in her extremities, poor concentration, memory loss, fatigue, headaches, and eye infections, plunged into a downward spiral of illness when her HMO's available physicians, inexperienced in dealing with Lyme, put the young teenager on steroids.

By the time she was admitted to the hospital, the child was nearly comatose, and "the only part of her body she could move was her right arm," says Marie. "I feel very strongly that my daughter would not have become so ill if my health group had some doctors more knowledgeable about Lyme disease or could have referred me to someone outside the group. Thank God I finally found a doctor who can not only treat my daughter, but because he has been diagnosed with Lyme himself, understands the disease. She.is getting better, but it's a long physical and emotional process, as well as a financial burden.

"Now many insurance companies are deciding how long a person should be on antibiotics, not the doctor. Does that make sense? We need to get off our soft denials that 'this will never happen to me' and do something, because this is affecting whole families."

Since the positive aspect of low medical costs through HMOs is derived from strict cost-containment practices and case managers who are paid to deny claims, and thereby save the company money, Lyme disease, with its potentially expensive and long treatment schedule, presents a major problem.

Chicago attorney Judee Gallagher, former counsel to the Illinois State Medical Society's Office of Contractual Services, has been repeatedly called upon to give advice regarding insurance and HMO coverage and liabilities. In an article for *Physician's Management*, she referred to the fact that, increasingly, HMOs are being cited as defendants in malpractice cases but have averted unfavorable verdicts if they can show that the physicians involved agreed in advance that the HMO's cost-containment actions and payment denials would not affect medical care.

Clinicians who are knowledgeable regarding Lyme disease would most likely not agree to such absolute payment restrictions, which would also restrict effective medical care, so, once again, the onus is on the medical consumer to beware.

MAKING YOUR INSURANCE PAY

Prophylactically, the best advice is to be sure you understand your health insurance policy and to review it periodically as family situations change. Most of us get those policy booklets and throw them into a file cabinet or drawer until we are in a desperate or litigious situation. Review the following:

- How much is your deductible? Is it per illness, per person, per year, or per family?
- What benefits are specifically covered? Look for mention of home care.
- What benefits are excluded? Generally, anything not specifically mentioned as a benefit is excluded.
- What is the lifetime maximum the plan will pay? What is the maximum it will pay for each illness?
- Under what conditions can the insurer cancel your plan?
- Are there limits on the types of services that are of interest to you? What are the limits on preexisting conditions?

If you have been diagnosed with disseminated Lyme and your physician recommends continued treatment but your insurance company refuses to continue coverage, the best advice given by the experts is "Don't give up!" Of major assistance is the journal that I recommended you keep (see chapter 3). Continued documentation of the illness, symptoms, treatment, and reactions to treatment provides you with supporting evidence with which to fight.

Protest vigorously, using all available procedures dictated by both your insurance company and your state. Exhaust all your options under your contract and make copies of everything in case your file "gets misplaced."

If appealing an insurance company decision, stay on top of it. Do not let weeks pass before following up on the course of your case. Continue to document your actions, the people you spoke with at the company, and the elapsed time involved, in addition to any reactions to stopping medication, if that becomes financially necessary. Ask your physician to send a strongly worded letter to the company stating that its action/inaction is impacting on the health of the patient. This may get the attention of the medical director, bypassing the clerical personnel who are handling routine claims.

Become politically active through a support group or by contacting your state legislators and holding them accountable. Remember, you may be sick, but those elected officials *work for you*. Give them a job to do!

Do not give up—you are not alone. If necessary, seek the outside support (this includes the media) of those who have experience in fighting for insurance claims and make your voice heard. Our political structure is such that you will be more successful if you can demonstrate support in numbers, and this will, in turn, provide your legislators with credibility to press your demands among their colleagues.

The injustice against Lyme patients by some members of the insurance industry is not going to be "cured" by anyone *but* Lyme patients and their advocates. The fight must be continued on a higher plane if families who are already struggling on so many fronts are to be able to enjoy paid treatment until they are well.

15.

Supportive Therapy or Sham?

"The doctor of the future will give no medicine but will interest his patients in the care of the human frame, in diet, and in the cause and prevention of disease."

—Thomas A. Edison

Gerald had been on antibiotics for Lyme disease for fifteen months when his chiropractor placed him on a definitive program of aerobic exercise, nutritional supplements, and acupuncture therapy. Within six weeks, Gerald was finally off medication and feeling healthier than he had in more than two years.

■ In California, ads promising a Lyme cure through meditation were published in a number of periodicals. The meditation course cost Elise $150. She said the only difference it made in her life was that she was $150 poorer and ashamed at having been taken as a fool.

■ In one tiny Atlantic Seaboard town, a man who holds no major certifications sells a serum marketed for Lyme disease patients. Since the serum is not a drug and he makes no promises, he is untouched by the law. But respectable local practitioners of holistic therapies and traditional physicians continually have to warn patients away from this man.

■ Most people laugh when confronted with vignettes about snake oil salesmen trying to persuade an innocent audience that the product they hawk will relieve their heartburn, cure their warts, give them fresh breath, and enhance their sexual performance. Yet those same people, in the midst of a chronic, painful, and debilitating illness like Lyme disease, can fall for a modern version of the snake oil pitch that promises pain relief and revived good health. These victims and others in the United States will spend whatever it takes, but they are the ones who wind up "taken," to the tune of approximately $40 billion per year.

There *are* some legitimate supportive therapies available for the relief of Lyme disease symptoms. They are designed to boost the body's own immune system or to recapture the strength lost from extensive illness and antibiotic therapy. The trick is learning to distinguish them from the sham therapies that abound.

MEDICAL CONSUMER, BEWARE!

For most of us who are plunged into the world of Lyme disease, the whole medical arena is like a trip to Mars. We are suddenly learning a new lingo, dealing with alien professionals, and navigating new waters—all the while feeling less than well, either physically, emotionally, or both.

We are prime targets for those who are disreputable and looking to make a quick buck off desperate people. The primary thing to remember is that *there is no quick fix for Lyme disease.*

Using that as a measuring stick, the medical consumer must be on the alert for:

• *Any remedy billed as a "cure."* There is no such thing at this time. If there were, you can bet that major companies would be advertising, producing, and disseminating it worldwide with the blessings of reputable clinicians and researchers.

• *Remedies available only through mail order or one source, or those that contain "secret ingredients."* This should make you suspicious immediately. Furthermore, remember that there is no "cure" for Lyme disease.

• *Doctors who advertise on billboards or in other splashy media.* Often, these doctors present case history testimonials but little in the way of research or substance. They rely on personality and advertising instead of solid therapeutic procedures and care.

• *Pseudo–Lyme disease hot lines.* Some hot lines truly provide solid information and referral services—if they're backed by a reputable nonprofit organization (i.e., the Lyme Disease Network). Some, however, are funded by companies seeking to be paid for such referrals, and may, in fact, give you the name of only one doctor—possibly the one who started the hot line. You should not pay for simple information. Call your local Lyme support group or hospital as an alternative if a call to a "hot line" seems bogus.

• *Practitioners of any sort who encourage total dependence upon them for your wellness.* Whether from the medical mainstream or from alternative medical therapies, the reputable physician will assist you to independent wellness. Anyone encouraging dependence is more interested in your pocketbook than in your health.

Traditionally, medical doctors have concerned themselves only with the pathology of illness, treatment of the patient's symptoms, and resolution of the signs of disease. Today, many of those who are treating Lyme disease—itself out of the mainstream disease path—recognize that medical science does not have all the answers and that adjunctive therapies, including new ways of eating, exercising, and reducing stress, may be just as important to the patient's recovery as the antibiotics prescribed.

Throw into the equation the success of medical treatments from other cultures, the need to treat the total person since Lyme disease is a multisystemic infection, and the desire and need for patients to take an active role in the process, and you have an approach to Lyme disease that is best termed "multimodal therapy."

LYME DISEASE REHABILITATION

Dr. Joseph Burrascano, of Long Island, New York, has been treating Lyme disease patients since the mid-1980s, although he says he has suffered with it since his own teenage years. He is a physician who has crossed that researcher-clinician barrier—as involved in research as most academics, yet treating a battalion of Lyme patients from an assortment of states across the country. His treatment procedures are based upon years of studying, recommending, refining, and practicing what he preaches.

"Those with long-standing Lyme end up in poor physical condition. Even with successful treatment of the Lyme infection, they will not return to normal unless they take an active role in personal rehabilitation," says Burrascano, who also serves on the medical advisory board to the Lyme Disease Foundation.

In the later stages of Lyme, muscles may spasm and atrophy; the heart muscle suffers; the joints, nerves, and liver are negatively affected; and the patient's overall stamina and immune system suffer. As a result, Lyme patients become weak, tired, and are at increased risk for heart attack and diabetes.

Burrascano maintains that physical therapy, particularly aerobics, has an important role in the patient's recovering his or her health and that, particularly with late-stagers, this therapy should be very individualized.

"One hundred percent of those who went into an aggressive rehabilitation program got better. It has a positive impact on reversing the effects of Lyme disease. I usually recommend that a patient begin slowly, and that immediately after exercising, they take a very hot bath and then nap. As the weeks go by, they won't need the nap and will gradually increase their level of activity."

Apart from the gradual strengthening of the overall body system, another reason that aerobics works for the Lyme patient is that it increases the blood flow and body temperature—a setting in which the spirochete cannot thrive.

"Diet also plays an important role," says Burrascano. "This is the time for the very best of health habits. I recommend light, low-fat food, with high-quality nutritional value, absolute abstention from alcohol, elimination of caffeine, and if applicable, a serious commitment to weight loss and cessation of smoking."

If your doctor is not well versed in nutrition beyond the customary "take a multiple vitamin" admonition, then you should seek out the assistance of a nutritional counselor for a program designed specifically for your needs.

An increasing number of doctors treating Lyme are educating themselves in nutritional therapies, or even referring their patients to other practitioners who, as an adjunct to antibiotic therapy, treat the whole person with the goal of strengthening the body to both fight off infection and reclaim its autonomy.

CHIROPRACTIC AND KINESIOLOGY

Mention the word "stress" to most people and they will immediately think of a weekend with unfavorite relatives, a job deadline, or financial or relationship problems. This is emotional stress, but doctors look at three other types of stressors, including physical, biochemical, and thermal.

Lyme disease patients suffer all four kinds of stress, yet antibiotic therapy addresses only the biochemical, and in doing so, causes further chemical stress to the body. For that reason, many Lyme patients are finding that chiropractic, kinesiology, and acupuncture—all of which are designed to realign the body's various energy systems—have not only provided relief of symptoms, but also assisted in boosting the body's immune system.

Dr. Edward Burstein is one of only 117 Diplomates of the International College of Applied Kinesiology worldwide. The founder of Berkeley Heights Chiropractic Center, in a Lyme-endemic area of New Jersey, he is a board-certified teacher and has lectured at numerous hospitals on immune, autoimmune, and chronic degenerative diseases. He is also seeing an increasing number of Lyme patients.

"Lyme disease seems to attack the weakest systems in a person's body. We see many, many people with Lyme, and every single person is different," says Burstein. "We need to tune up each person to as high a functioning level as possible.

"When the body is in a stressed state, many physiological changes take place. Blood pressure goes up, digestion slows, and muscles tense—all of the body's systems are on alert to deal with the stress. Continued distress is harmful because the body becomes exhausted from working overtime. If the stress is emotional or biochemical in nature, and continues, the resistance phase begins; the body attempts to adapt to the stress. This phase can go on for a long time and eventually the body weakens.

"The last phase is exhaustion or burnout," says Burstein.

"The body no longer has the energy to contain the stress and begins to break down. Expressed as chronic fatigue, this phase is probably the most universal in our society."

This breakdown of the body's natural defenses complicates both the treatment for and the recovery from Lyme disease in that it can mask other problems. Harry, a fifty-year-old designer and avid jogger, was in a disseminated stage of Lyme before he was diagnosed. By that time, he could hardly get out of bed. Still symptomatic after fourteen months on antibiotics, he sought an adjunctive therapy. It was discovered that not only did he have a parasite in his intestine, but there was mercury in his system as well, which contributed to his swollen knees. Two months of treatment cleared up both problems, and his body began to reclaim its strength and his Lyme symptoms diminished.

The emphasis, once again, is on a multimodal approach to attacking Lyme. Straight medical treatment may not relieve all symptoms, and straight chiropractic may not either. If you are inclined to employ an adjunctive therapy, you should look for a medical doctor, osteopath, or chiropractor who practices applied kinesiology. This is a system that not only evaluates the body's structural, chemical, and mental aspects, but also utilizes nutrition, diet, acupressure (similar to acupuncture but without needles), and exercise to revive the total person.

A reputable practitioner will perform a number of noninvasive diagnostic medical tests before recommending a specific treatment path.

HOMEOPATHY

Another version of natural healing is homeopathy, which was begun in the early 1800s by German physician Samuel Hahnemann. His beliefs that "like cures like" and that medicines become more potent as they are diluted have given rise to a whole field of noninvasive therapy that has ardent detractors as well as ardent followers—including the British royal family, which has had a homeopathic doctor on staff since the time of Queen Victoria.

Much of homeopathy includes solid nutrition and life-style practices, and for those doctors like David Frerking, of Tavares, Florida, who are seeing an increasing number of Lyme patients, it is part of a multimodal attack on the disease.

"My approach is not to treat Lyme specifically, but to treat the entire body after performing a number of diagnostic tests," says Frerking, a member of the Board of Chiropractic Diagnosis and Preventive Medicine. "Traditional medicine says we must control the body; chiropractic philosophy says our bodies know how to be healthy and control themselves. When that's interfered with, the body's ability to function breaks down.

"Antibiotics given for Lyme disease push the organism into the cells. Homeopathics draws it out into the bloodstream where the body can find it. The substances used in homeopathy are diluted to stimulate the body to enhance its own response to fight off infection."

■ The important things to remember when seeking adjunctive therapies for Lyme disease are caution and common sense. Many feel, however, that they don't know where to turn for adequate information and assume that, if something was important for the public to know, the health department would be the first to tell them. They assume too much.

16.

Practical Prevention and the Public Health

"Were it not for AIDS, Lyme disease would be the number one threat to the nation as an infectious disease."

—Dr. Anita Curran, former director, New York State Department of Health

Berkley Bedell, a former congressman and entrepreneur from Iowa, thought he was out for a day of fun when he pushed his small boat through tall grass at the edge of a Virginia lake about five years ago and received a tick bite. The health problems that followed, due to Lyme disease, forced his retirement from Congress.

■ Spring and fall are prime seasons for school field trips, outdoor sports, and nature walks. Doctors in Lyme-endemic areas are beginning to track increased reports of tick bites and Lyme symptoms in children during these two critical times of year.

■ Public health officials from across the country complain that budget cutbacks leave little funding for the protection of the public from contagious infectious diseases, let alone dollars for education and prevention of Lyme.

■ Ovid, that ancient Roman who held some minor government positions before retiring to write poetry, might not have anticipated Lyme disease when he penned his often quoted and paraphrased line "The best defense is a good offense," but it has become the battle cry of those in the Lyme arena. The surest "cure" for Lyme disease is protection and education, and this must occur in three areas: your own person, home, and community.

Because Lyme disease is a very real environmental hazard and has a negative impact on the health of an area, people are beginning to become paranoid about participating in activities they formerly enjoyed. Many have given up camping, hiking, jogging, fishing, hunting, or even picnicking, especially in Lyme-endemic areas. Parents have forbidden their children to go out and play in the yard, go on school field trips to recreational areas, or leave the house unless covered from head to toe with clothing. And some health department officials attempt to walk a fine line between animal rights activists who protest deer hunting and frightened citizens who would like to wipe out any population of animals that might carry the infected ticks.

The problem with all of these anxious approaches is that they are treating the symptom and not the problem. Like the citizen who puts bars on his windows and does not go outside because of an increase in crime in the neighborhood, some citizens are becoming prisoners in their own homes and offices because of the danger of Lyme disease.

The problem is the infected tick and the solution is eradication. *This* is where a major emphasis of education and protection must be—not on the elimination of activities. Once again, the solution is available, but it is up to each of us to implement it personally and demand its implementation on community and statewide levels.

PERSONAL PROTECTION

Most of us who have had any contact with Lyme disease, either personally or through the media, are familiar with the warning to wear long pants tucked into socks, long-sleeved shirts, gloves, and goggles, if possible. While this is ideal, and may discourage a tick from getting to one's skin, the image of having to bundle up during hot weather spells, when tick infestation is highest, may have a reverse effect on the public's motivation. Shorts, T-shirts, and bathing suits are here to stay, so other precautions against tick bite also need to be taken.

The following guidelines for personal protection against tick bites should be followed particularly in those areas in which Lyme is endemic and especially during the months of May through October.

- Don't walk barefoot or in open sandals outside. In Lyme-endemic areas, even short grass can harbor infected ticks.
- Since feet, ankles, and legs are primary points of contact, do wear long pants if walking through woods or tall grasses. Likewise, a hat is advisable if you are going to be in the woods or tall vegetation.
- Use a repellent on exposed skin or on clothing or camping gear if outdoor activities are going to be prolonged. Since repellents on skin are potentially neurotoxic, spraying something like Permanone on the clothes and equipment may be better tolerated.
- Wear light-colored clothing so ticks will be more visible upon inspection.
- Check yourself every several hours during a long outing,

and even more thoroughly upon returning home, prefera-
bly while you are still outside. Remember to look in those
areas where ticks like to hide: the base of the neck, waist-
bands and/or brassieres, under arms, behind the knees,
around ankles, in underwear.

- Take any clothing worn and throw it into the dryer for
  fifteen minutes on high heat. This will kill any ticks on
  the clothes. (Ticks have been known to live underwater
  for days, so putting the clothes in the washing machine
  will be ineffective.)

- Shower and brush hair thoroughly to discourage the attachment of any ticks.

- If you go outside to carry firewood into the house, consider using a repellent-sprayed carrier instead of holding
  the wood against your body.

- If camping, spray your equipment and tent with an effective repellent (see below) that lasts for up to forty-eight
  hours. When changing clothes, seal those that have been
  worn in a plastic bag until you can get them home to put
  in the dryer.

- Hunters and trappers should hang animal carcasses away
  from human activity for at least twelve hours so that ticks
  have a chance to drop off. In order to prevent the ticks
  from simply dropping off and crawling away, place a
  bucket of water with a concentration of liquid bleach
  directly under the carcass to kill falling ticks. If the carcass
  is being dressed in the field, it is advisable to wear rubber
  gloves to minimize chances of infection.

- Inspect your children daily for ticks and/or teach them to
  inspect themselves, particularly in "private" areas of their
  bodies.

- If you do find a tick, do not panic. Also, do not use a
  cigarette, petroleum jelly, nail polish, kerosene, or a match
  to remove it. This will only cause the tick to inject more

"poison" into your system. Grasp the tick with fine tweezers, as close to the skin as possible, and pull gently, straight out. You can then place the tick in a small plastic bag or other container with a blade of grass or some moist cotton and take it to your doctor or health department for testing. If you live in a Lyme-endemic area, contact your internist and report the tick bite to him.

USING REPELLENTS

Ideally, an effective vaccine against Lyme disease would be a part of childhood inoculations, or at least as common as flu shots. Although Yale University and the University of New Mexico are both working toward that end, it may be years before such a form of protection is available to the public. Until then, the best method of protection is the use of repellents.

Few people would advocate spraying chemicals needlessly on the human body, but it is generally accepted that the dangers of Lyme disease warrant the added protection of safe tick repellents. The most effective repellent that can be safely applied to the skin contains a component known as DEET.

Developed originally for use in the military during the 1950s, DEET is commonly used now by more than an estimated 200 million people a year. A five-year compilation of data from the American Association of Poison Control Centers showed products containing DEET to be relatively safe, and it is approved for use by the Environmental Protection Agency (EPA) as well.

Two of the more popular and effective products manufactured with DEET include the Repel line from Wisconsin Pharmacal Company, which produces several products in varying strengths for specific purposes, and Deep Woods Off.

It is important to remember that the manufacturer's instructions should be carefully read and followed prior to use. There is no need to "take a bath" in the repellent, and it should be applied in a well-ventilated area. Inhaling fumes or overspraying can result in adverse reactions, and repellent should never be sprayed over cut or broken skin.

A repellent that was tested by the military, particularly in Saudi Arabia, and found to be 100 percent effective in killing and repelling ticks is permethrin. It is commercially available in an aerosol spray under the names Permanone, from Innovative Labs, Jackson, Wisconsin, or Duranon, from Coulston International, of Easton, Pennsylvania. A single application to clothing or equipment is effective for up to two days. Remember that safe application consists of spraying the clothing while it is *off* the body, then allowing it to dry in a well-ventilated area before wearing.

A newly released formula, Permethrin Tick Repellent, is supposed to offer protection for up to two weeks. The only drawback to Permanone is that it is not available in all states.

MAKE YOUR HOME UNINVITING

Making one's home a castle usually involves investing hours and dollars in landscaping, ornamental walks and walls, and lawn maintenance. Unfortunately, not only do humans find shrubs, hanging vines, and trees inviting, so do ticks.

In a CDC study of four hundred properties in upstate New York, several common factors were revealed. According to Dr. Durland Fish, associate professor and director of the Lyme Disease Center for New York Medical College:

• Tick infestation was seven times higher in those areas that were unmaintained (i.e., woods, borders, or "natural" landscaping).

- Stone walls are favorite places for ticks to congregate, so humans should avoid sitting on or working around them during those times of year when nymphal ticks are active.

- Ticks love ornamental shrubs.

- Insecticide application of Sevin (carbaryl), Dursban (chlorpyrifos), and permethrin was 97 percent effective in controlling ticks for the entire nymphal season. Although the permethrin worked the best, it is not available in all states. Both Sevin and Dursban are commonly used, both on lawns and in a number of pet products, with good safety records. The granular form of the insecticides was more effective on lawns, which are not critical habitats for wildlife.

Sensitive to public criticism of the use of pesticides, Fish says, "You have a choice between being exposed to insecticides or Lyme disease. It's your decision.

"Remember, it's not the ticks that you find that are the ones likely to give you trouble. They are the failures, the losers. The successful ticks are the ones you don't see."

There are several other home-based strategies that can be employed to reduce the risk of tick attraction. One method is to increase the lawn size, pushing trees, ornamentals, and hedges away from the house. Since open lawn has the lowest rate of tick infestation across the board, cutting back on the number of shade trees, particularly those close to the house, will reduce your risk.

It is wise to locate children's sandboxes and swing sets in open, sunny areas rather than shady ones. A large beach umbrella raised during sandbox play will protect little ones from the sun's harmful rays, yet allow you to keep the unit in an area unattractive to ticks.

Finally, go after the mouse population, which serves as an important host for ticks. Not only are the mice carriers during the summer months, but when the weather turns cold they tend to run for nice warm houses—bringing their ticks with them.

Aiming to control the ticks that feed on mice, Harvard University researchers developed Damminix. This is cotton soaked with permethrin and packed in biodegradable tubes that are placed around a specific property. The mice collect the cotton, take it back to their nests for building material, and kill ticks in the process. This has been shown to be effective, but it must be widely used in a given geographic location to have a major impact.

Personal protection and the regular trimming of one's lawn are an excellent start to preventing Lyme disease. These methods, however, will not do the job unless we bring both the problem and the solution to the attention of those in our cities and states who have the power to implement important community protection programs.

COMMUNITY PROTECTION: A TAXPAYER'S RIGHT

Many citizens only come in contact with their state's health department via unsafe restaurants, school health rules, or travel plans that require immunizations. Good medical consumers, however, should know what their health department is doing in the areas of environmental hazards, disease control, and education. After all, they are paying for these services through tax dollars.

As a parent and a citizen, I am concerned about our landscaped park areas, particularly those near shopping and historical sites, where we would stroll leisurely. I am concerned about school and community fields (typically bordered by woods and natural vegetation), where my children play soccer and field hockey, fly kites, or watch sporting events and outdoor concerts.

These, in particular, are frequented by deer and populated by ticks.

And, although health officials are faced with severe budget cutbacks, increasing responsibilities, and new infectious threats, Lyme disease education and protection can and should be a priority. This is especially true in the face of this worsening epidemic and the possible legal ramifications of someone's acquiring Lyme in a known endemic area on an unprotected public site. The claim by county health departments that there is little room in the budget for additional programs is a valid one, but a number of public health officials who recognize the importance and impact of the growing Lyme epidemic have managed to implement extensive programs through the use of organizational skills and interested volunteers. A perfect example of such a program is the Lyme Disease Project of Stamford, Connecticut.

Dr. Andrew McBride is a large man with an easygoing manner, perhaps developed from being the oldest of twelve siblings. He is also a physician who has seen it all. Former commissioner of public health for Washington, D.C., and senior vice president for advocacy for the Children's Hospital, he brought to Connecticut a background that included administering multimillion-dollar budgets and experience with issues ranging from addictions and child abuse to community preventive medicine policies. But one of his biggest challenges came with his position as director of health for the city of Stamford, where, as the new kid in the department, he was besieged with reports of Lyme disease and tick infestation.

"If you really want to get something done quickly, have your director of health personally answer the telephones for one day," he said, chuckling. "You find out what's happening in the community and where the needs are."

He found the need for education on Lyme disease was reaching desperate proportions, but there was no program and no funding was available. Undaunted, he turned to his staff and the community at large. "It is a matter of prioritizing," he says. "It's the public that drives a program like this, the public and a staff of volunteers. The people have to be committed and competent to make it work.

"One of the first things we did was to get the labs to begin testing ticks. Every state has some lab facility within its government structure. We found that tick identification was one of the more powerful tools for tracking where the illness was spreading. The incidence of infected ticks showed us that we were in an endemic area. If a county doesn't have an agricultural station that can handle some of these responsibilities, it can assign people to do a study to get a quantity of ticks for evaluation. Just tell people where to send them—the people will respond, believe me. And something important to remember is that just because a person brings in a tick which is not infected is not an assurance that they haven't been bitten by another one that is."

Integral to a Lyme disease education project is a cooperative relationship with the local media, says McBride. Approach the editors of local newspapers, develop a relationship with science or community reporters, and don't forget any local radio or television stations. This is a partnership that can help each party.

Utilizing various health department personnel and volunteers, a mass education effort was then launched. This included the following:

• *School systems.* Since teachers are concerned about field trips as well as seeking out new avenues of learning, and kids are very aware of health threats, schools are a primary target for information. This included encouragement of student science projects and reports, letters to parents and administrators, information posters on Lyme, and the thorough education of school nurses.

- *Libraries.* The health department hit these with posters, brochures, and exhibits.

- *Parks and beaches.* On-site educational programs were held, and posters and brochures were made a part of the site.

- *Local physicians.* Educational presentations as well as letters and informational brochures were distributed.

- *Health fairs.* Booths and presentations were set up to offer information to families, corporations, and hospitals, and to encourage community involvement.

- *A speakers' bureau.* Continuing educational presentations are made to county and city employees, utility workers, corporations, and other outdoor organizations and workers.

McBride realizes that not all health departments are sympathetic to the Lyme disease situation for various reasons, but says that should not stop the public from taking action.

"If you are turned away by your health department, seek out a sympathetic and knowledgeable internist or infectious disease specialist to assist in setting up a program. Every state has some facility already in place that people can utilize as a satellite. Sometimes it's a medical school or a medical center. Find out who is in charge of infectious diseases and talk to that person.

"The politics of public health would tend to downplay anything that would upset the status quo. Public health service is traditionally a conservative wing," says McBride. "This is why it is important to have those numbers—of ticks, infected people, actual cases. It sets up some credibility. The public health departments set the tone for local physicians, and I feel they have a responsibility to educate those physicians. If the physician gets a signal to either worry or not worry about a particular matter, that impression can last a long time. In the meantime, new facts may come to light that need to be passed on. This is an ongoing process. And a very important one."

■ As has been said by those toiling in the Lyme field, the ultimate responsibility for education and activism is in the hands of those affected by the disease. Enlightened health officials and doctors can do only so much: the driving force for change must be the public. This realization has fueled the formation of growing numbers of support groups, coalitions, and political entities.

17.

Support and Activism: A Vital Link

"To see what is right and not to do it is want of courage."

—Confucius, *Analects*

Prior to the Civil War, one of the first organized support networks was established in the United States. It was called the Underground Railroad. Although it was neither a railroad nor underground, it provided runaway slaves with information, contacts, and a helping hand to freedom. And it provided more; it let them know that they were not alone in their plight and that there were many who would risk their own safety and livelihood to do the right thing.

Today, another type of "underground railroad" is in effect across the country, and its mission is not terribly unlike its predecessor's. Along this network, Lyme disease patients can find information, names of doctors who are brave enough to treat them, sympathy, and encouragement in their flight to freedom from a disease that can enslave both the mind and the body. And they, too, are finding more than they expected.

In order to be heard above the din of needy voices and the kaleidoscope of demands pelting our nation's medical establishment and its lawmakers, these Lyme disease patients, doctors, and advocates are developing networks of political activism. From California to Wisconsin to New England to Florida, support groups have been activated, coalitions formed, independent projects undertaken, and legislation written, all in the name of freedom from Lyme. And as surely as the Underground Railroad crystallized the polarity of the country regarding slavery, the exploding Lyme disease movement promises to forge a new look at health care and patients' rights in the face of massive bureaucratic denial and lethargy.

FINDING SUPPORT, FINDING SANITY

They walk in gingerly the first time, some shuffling slowly, some leaning on canes, family members, or walkers. Most are desperate—ill, depressed, financially strained, and frustrated over a medical enigma that has infected the whole family's psyche. And what they find at the Lyme support group meeting is more than they had hoped for: reassurance that they are not alone or crazy (despite the fact that several doctors might have told them they were); education about this complex disease and avenues for treatment; and contact with others of every race, creed, and color who can offer practical methods of dealing with annoying symptoms that well-meaning but inexperienced doctors cannot provide.

Whether you're speaking with Richard Goldman or Linda Carrizales in Florida, Laura Ames in California, Kathy Cavert in Missouri, or Lora Mermin in Wisconsin, you hear that their reasons for starting a support group were the same: anger and frustration. Anger at members of the medical profession for abdicating their responsibility to teach the public about this disease and then reacting with arrogance when confronted by continual illness; and frustration over the isolation the illness imposes, the loss of control over one's body systems, and the emotional havoc it wreaks.

Betty Gross is a petite spitfire who exudes energy and confidence. A mother of four (two of whom are doctors) and a grandmother, she was a veteran of years of volunteer work with Girl Scouts, Twins Clubs, and special interest groups in her Westchester, New York, community when she was hit with Lyme disease. Suddenly, folding a basket of laundry not only had to be planned, it exhausted her so badly that she needed a three-hour nap to recover. Searching for information regarding this strange illness that was sweeping through her community in 1988, she found little available. What she found were afflicted neighbors who would call and say, "Am I going to live through this?"

She turned to the county health department and volunteered her services to get information out to the community and the doctors. She involved the newspapers and local service groups. Each outreach brought a flood of response and need. After attending a leadership training course for support groups, she placed a small blurb in the local newspaper about the formation of a group for those involved in Lyme disease.

"We had to change our location twice even before that first meeting because the telephone calls in response to the newspaper ad were overwhelming," says Betty. "Finally, Reverend Charles Colwell of the Saint Barnabas Episcopal Church just told me to take over the whole church and it's a good thing he did."

More than seventy people packed the charming white colonial church that evening in 1988, and the first Lyme support group in the nation was established. Today, the Westchester group's monthly newsletter has an active mailing list of more than three hundred names, while another several hundred fluctuate in attendance and participation. Still under the leadership of Betty Gross, the group has been responsible for staging informative conferences and seminars on Lyme disease for both doctors and the public, disseminating information on Lyme, setting up an information hot line (manned by Betty Monday through Friday from 10 A.M. to 4 P.M.), and interceding for numerous patients who have been unfairly treated by employers, schools, insurance companies, and doctors.

"No one can amply gauge when you 'hit bottom' in Lyme disease because it's different for each person," says Betty. "No one has an idea of how Lyme is going to twist and mangle your existence until it happens. People have to plumb the depths of themselves to deal with this. When a person contracts Lyme, their whole family becomes infected. When it is a child, other children in the family become invisible under the impact of this disease. And Lyme makes people paranoid because of the reactions of those around them. We've had a number of professionals who didn't want their colleagues to know they had Lyme disease because the public hears syphilis and Lyme mentioned in the same sentence and they mentally connect the two diseases and avoid the Lyme patient.

"Confidentiality is what a support group has going for it. As a leader, you become privy to people's confidences, a private surrendering of one's self as they share their feelings, their agonies, and their worries. If anyone thinks they would like to start a group, they must realize that they have to be able to keep these confidences locked up inside—or don't do it."

Here is some further advice for those wishing to start a support group:

• Support groups need to be conduits of information. Evaluate the doctors in the area and attempt to involve the enlightened ones. Then, when the confidence of the group leaders is stronger, invite the other doctors in the area.

• Begin with your local health department, but don't rely solely on it. Develop a relationship with the local media and exchange information.

• Bring in speakers from pharmaceutical companies dealing with Lyme, legislators, and physicians, but leave time at meetings for people to network and share their feelings and experiences. This is an important aspect of the support group because it lets people know that they are not as isolated as they think, either in their struggles or their emotional strain—and that there is hope.

"We had one woman who spent twenty-nine days mustering the strength to get to the meeting, and then took a week to recover from the strain of getting there," says Betty. "But it was that important to her. A support group is more special than a fraternity or sorority because the Lyme experience pushes a button of intimacy; this is how Lyme affects people and how they talk to each other. The wellspring of friendships that form is incredible to see as whole families help each other get through this thing."

At least Lyme disease was acknowledged as a problem in upstate New York. Kathy Cavert, in Independence, Missouri, and Linda Carrizales, in South Florida, were fighting the popular perception that the disease didn't exist in their states. Yet with the inception of their support groups, patients flocked to meetings hungering for information and contact with others who were experiencing the same frustrations.

"This whole idea of Lyme hysteria is just the reverse," says Kathy, a registered nurse who has specialized in psychotherapy. Infected with Lyme since the late 1980s, she is now disabled but struggles to publish newsletters and was responsible for a national survey of doctors and patients to compile an accurate list of Lyme symptoms. "There is so much denial going on, not only with governments but with the patients themselves. People will justify all their symptoms by saying, 'Oh, I slept wrong, I'm under stress, I'm at that age when my body should be falling apart anyway' (this from people in their thirties and forties!). People have to be educated so they can get well.

"This disease isn't hitting the couch potatoes of the country who sit in front of the television drinking beer," says Kathy. "It's hitting the most active, brightest *doers*, and it is forcing them to have to reframe their whole existence in order to survive."

From Broward County, Florida, Linda Carrizales has to reassure those who call her from across the country that yes, Lyme does exist in Florida, and then outline the steps they need to take to obtain the proper diagnosis and treatment. Afflicted with Lyme during her teens, she had the disease for thirteen years before it was diagnosed as the source of her continual health problems. Her group has staged informative seminars for doctors and patients at South Florida hospitals, but the strain of juggling patients, information, and people's pain is wearing, she says.

"A large part of what we do is information and support, and this becomes a full-time job. I would tell anyone wanting to start a group to make sure you have help, backup of some kind, and if you can get informed doctors involved that's even better. Part of our problem here in Florida is that we have hundreds upon hundreds of people infected and the doctors don't know anything about it; patients have to go out of state for treatment."

Lora Mermin, in Madison, Wisconsin, experienced the same type of situation when she was first infected in 1987. By 1988, a small ad placed in the local newspaper brought a half dozen people to an informational meeting of what is now the Lyme Resource Group of Madison and South Central Wisconsin. Inspired by the hunger for information, Lora formed the Lyme Disease Education Project and combined informative issues of Lyme support group newsletters from across the country and published them under one cover. She, too, recognizes the need for people to reach out and make contact with those who can understand the Lyme experience. "We have some people who drive for two hours to get to our meetings. People are eager to talk; they need to know that they aren't crazy and that there is help available to them."

A number of the older and more active support groups have been the birthplaces of monthly newsletters that provide information and hope to thousands across the country (see appendix B), and a few more have made the transition into the national arena.

The Lyme Disease Network, established by Carol and Bill Stolow in reaction to their young daughters' infection with Lyme, has recently moved from serving the state of New Jersey to linking support groups across the country. In addition to serving as a conduit for information and as a link for widely spread groups, the Stolows are establishing a special information line strictly for physicians across the country who want to know more about Lyme disease. Carol, an education supervisor for Rutgers University, and Bill, a marketing manager, have talked local milk companies into putting Lyme information on their cartons to reach people right in their homes.

Joe Burke, a former scientific computer programmer and head of a support group for chronic fatigue syndrome (CFS) sufferers, found after years of physical deterioration that what he had was Lyme disease, not chronic fatigue. His American Lyme Disease Alliance concentrates on presenting the most current medical and psychosocial information to both patients and doctors across the country.

"The terms 'chronic fatigue syndrome' and 'Lyme disease' have been used interchangeably by many physicians, and it is now a well-known fact that thousands upon thousands of Lyme sufferers have been misdiagnosed this way," says Burke, whose group also sponsors conferences and publications. For political and insurance reasons, many patients are diagnosed with CFS because the cost disparity in treating the two illnesses is so great. While Lyme, caused by a bacteria, can cost upwards of $50,000 a year to treat, CFS is caused by the Epstein-Barr virus and is untreatable. Patients are sometimes given antidepressants and told to get counseling. "And a number of patients are misdiagnosed simply because many doctors are just not well-educated in Lyme disease," says Burke. "To rectify this situation, patients should provide their doctors with the latest Lyme information available. These patients will, hopefully, be rewarded in return with more empathy and better treatment."

THE INDEPENDENT ACTIVISTS

Fred Lawson was just a fifteen-year-old Louisiana boy when he suffered such severe head trauma in an accident that he officially died. His experience as he traveled back to life, to the hospital room where his body lay, led him to the knowledge that he was put back on earth for a specific reason. After years of struggling to relearn the simplest speech and life skills, he was infected with Lyme disease.

Now in his fifties, Lawson, who resides in Leesburg, Florida, and is a sales manager for one of the country's largest repellent manufacturers, dedicates his life to providing support for those suffering with Lyme. This dedication has led him to organize a network of 250 volunteers to meet airplanes carrying Lyme patients from Florida to treatment in New York and New Jersey. It has led him to develop Lyme educational programs with former Rams player Jim Youngblood and to speak nationally on the subject. He has also talked suicidal Lyme patients off roofs and found doctors for those in remote areas.

"It's so important that people work together—not against each other—to beat this disease," he says. "I've seen the devastation Lyme disease can cause; I've seen the pain and suffering, and I've been through it myself and am still going through it. Just about the time you think you have a handle on it, it comes at you from a different direction. People in this country are extremely ill and they need help. I know that this is why I was put back on earth, and I'll do what little I can to educate people about Lyme."

Two Hollywood producers who were touched by Lyme have also moved into the educational arena by developing independent projects designed to educate both citizens and lawmakers.

When Neil Goldstein moved from Southern California to Pennsylvania five years ago, he found himself infected with Lyme disease and with nowhere to turn for information. He, along with Amy Jones, formed the Lyme Project of Hudson Valley. Initially set up to launch a multimodal attack on the problem, the project initiated epidemiological studies, produced public television programs, and established a support group. The project is now in the process of reorganization, and Goldstein says they are shooting for the involvement of area hospitals and medical personnel.

"There is no specialty in Lyme disease. We have to get people involved in their own health care so the doctors will be more aware of the problem and how to approach it."

Vincent Sorrentino's involvement with Lyme disease occurred when he was approached about filming a video to be shown to lawmakers in the New Jersey legislature who were trying to determine whether insurance companies should be mandated to continue coverage of their patients with Lyme. Although he had produced numerous documentaries on various human conditions, Lyme affected him so deeply that he formed Lyme Awareness Productions with several Lyme support groups for continued work in this area. Involved in producing the television docudrama about Lyme titled "The Hidden Epidemic," Sorrentino interviewed a number of children with the disease and walked away shaken. "On top of the incredible pain they endure, these kids have lost their friends, fallen behind in school, and seen their dreams disappear. It's very important that we do everything possible to bring awareness to the effects that Lyme disease is having on kids."

ACTIVIST GROUPS

When New York congressman George Hochbrueckner began talking about Lyme disease, many of his colleagues thought he was talking about something that afflicted citrus fruit. As one of the primary forces behind passage of a bill that would allocate nearly a million dollars for the protection from and treatment of Lyme disease in our armed forces overseas, and of another bill, cosponsored by Congressman Joseph Lieberman of Connecticut, proposing a national Lyme Awareness Week, he has served as the inspiration for many who want to move the Lyme battle into the political spotlight.

In early 1992, Governor Jim Florio of New Jersey approved the Governor's Lyme Advisory Council, the first such group in the nation, comprising a cross section of experts to make recommendations for combating the disease. Following closely was the formation of the New York Lyme Disease Coalition (New Jersey already had one), and similar moves in several other states, including Wisconsin, which began organizing their own coalitions to serve as umbrella organizations linking the diverse support groups for political clout.

Ken Fordyce, chairman of the New Jersey Governor's Advisory Council and longtime member of the New Jersey Lyme Disease Coalition, feels that organized, unified efforts are the only way anything will be accomplished in solving the Lyme puzzle. His group has immersed itself in everything from legislation to education to producing a position paper outlining the rights of patients and listing recommendations for action, which highlight the need for long-term treatment and drug studies.

"People need to become involved because nothing will be done unless they are," says Fordyce. "If AIDS hadn't come along, Lyme disease would be the hottest disease under discussion right now because, among other things, it's so chemically interesting. But getting to the heart of the problem goes back to territorial imperative—people stake out a position and then defend it to the death. Our job as medical consumers is to bombard them with the latest information available and push for action. We're talking about our lives here, and the lives of our children."

A number of support groups, foundations, alliances, and coalitions have formed to jump into the battle against Lyme disease. As recognition of the disease spreads, many more will be formed. One word of caution to the newly involved is necessary.

Any cause attracts the entire spectrum of human personality, from the reticent to the fanatic, from the educated to the ignorant, from the altruistic to the greedy. Lyme disease is no exception. The vast majority of organizations and foundations are reputable, but the wise medical consumer will ask some tough questions based on common sense before donating money or following a leader into battle.

Those organizations that ask for your donation, even on a well-publicized national level, should be able to provide you with an annual report of how the money is spent as well as references that should be checked out. You do not have to pay for referrals to doctors or groups; these are free through local support groups (see appendix A), newsletters (there is a legitimate charge for the publication itself), and independent hot lines (see appendices A and B).

Finally, educate yourself as to the nature of the disease and the political structure of the battle, rather than blindly joining under any banner proclaiming "Lyme." Remember, you can make a difference. You are the only one who *can* make a difference, but only if you join the fight as an informed medical consumer, not merely a passionate one.

18.
Conclusion: A Challenge to Fight

During the 1962 Cuban missile crisis between the United States and the Soviet Union, President John F. Kennedy received two conflicting communications from Soviet chairman Nikita Khrushchev. One contained terms that were acceptable, the other did not. Attorney General Robert Kennedy was credited with a diplomatic maneuver—later dubbed the "Trollope ploy," after a recurrent theme in Anthony Trollope's novels in which the girl interprets a squeeze of her hand as a proposal of marriage. Robert Kennedy's suggestion was to deal with the acceptable message only and to ignore the other. President Kennedy went on to accept Khrushchev's offer and then set forth his own ideas of what that offer really was.

There are many medical consumers who will maintain that their physicians, insurance companies, and health agencies are masters of Trollope's ploy when dealing with Lyme disease. These entities will accept those symptoms and statements that fit neatly into preconceived patterns and ignore others, substituting their own experience and ideas for the facts.

While this gambit may work in international negotiations, it subverts the doctor-patient relationship, delays or circumvents successful treatment, and contributes to the continued ill health of formerly talented and productive citizens.

Not too long ago there was a wonderful "Hagar the Horrible" comic strip that could have been inspired by a Lyme patient. The town's doctor has chased down the rotund Viking Hagar and his wife, Helga, and admonishes them: "You should trust doctors more. . . . Our first rule is: 'Do No Harm.' " Whereupon Helga turns to Hagar and comments, "It worries me that they'd need a *rule* to figure that out!"

Two basic medical tenets are: (1) patients want to get well, and (2) doctors want to heal. In dealing with Lyme disease, these two groups more than ever before are going to have to put aside traditional methodologies and attack the problem rather than each other. This can be accomplished through the following methods:

1. Citizens today must view themselves as medical consumers and take responsibility for both maintaining good health and for participating in their own medical treatment when ill.

2. Physicians need to keep an open mind—and open ears—when dealing with Lyme and other difficult diseases that may require more reliance on their own powers of deductive reasoning than on unreliable tests. Medicine is an art and a science. None of us can ignore the "art" aspect as we attempt to utilize the scientific principles.

3. Contracts outlining the principles of a therapeutic alliance should be signed by both the participating physician and the medical consumer prior to embarking on diagnosis and treatment of Lyme disease, thereby emphasizing the need for collaborative effort and setting the tone for a dynamic investigative relationship.

4. Doctors from both Lyme disease polarities need to put petty rivalries aside and work together to attack this illness. This natural competition is being utilized by both government and private institutions to ignore the growing problem of Lyme disease. The bottom line is: the patient loses. And with the rapid spread of this illness, the very doctors who downplay the dis-

ease's prevalence could find themselves on the patient's end of the tongue depressor.

5. Representatives from the American Medical Association and the American Bar Association should draw up guidelines governing disease protocols and malpractice insurance awards, so that the litigation process does not undermine the fair and equal practice of medicine. Further, the AMA should take a leadership role in educating the health insurance industry in this country, guaranteeing the American public the fair and equal coverage for which they have paid.

Finally, it is only through a unified commitment to good health education and medical practices, by our government agencies, our medical community, and our citizenry, that both doctors and patients can get on with the business of relieving pain and curing Lyme disease, thereby ensuring the continued leadership of the country.

Max Planck, the Nobel Prize–winning German physicist credited with laying the groundwork for the development of the quantum theory, knew what it was like to fly in the face of established scientific thought. "A new scientific truth does not triumph by convincing its opponents and making them see the light," he said, "but rather because its opponents eventually die, and a new generation grows up that is familiar with it."

Thousands of men, women, and children with Lyme disease cannot wait for the scientific and political foot-draggers to die before funding for research and treatment of this potent disease is made a priority. Too many of their own lives could be lost in the meantime.

Appendix A:
Support Groups, Resources, and Foundations

SUPPORT GROUPS BY STATE (AND CANADA)

AUTHOR'S NOTE: Every attempt has been made to present as current a list as possible, from a variety of sources. No attempt has been made to screen support groups or their leaders.

ARKANSAS
Fairfield Bay Lyme Support
  Group
Mary Alice Beer
Fairfield Bay, AR
(501) 884-3502

CALIFORNIA
Kern County Lyme/CFS Support
  Group
Helen Weygand
Bakersfield, CA
(805) 323-0649

Seaview Support Group
John Lushenko
Cazadero, CA
(707) 847-3445

Northern Central California
  LSG
Laura Lee Ames
Coalinga, CA
(209) 935-0914

Naval Warfare Assessment Cr.
  LSG
Frank Bartzatt
Corona, CA
(714) 736-4602

Central California LDSG
Mark Andrew and Richard
  Marshall
Fresno, CA
(no number available)

Lake County LDSG
Lakeside Community Hospital
Melanie McDougal
Lakeport, CA
(707) 263-5112

Lyme Borreliosis Network
June Casey
Oakland, CA
(510) 531-5357

Pacific Presbyterian Hospital
Holly Hebert
San Francisco, CA
(415) 923-3155

Santa Rosa LDSG
Betty Owens
Santa Rosa, CA
(707) 539-9395

Sonoma Valley Hospital LSG
Karen McDonald
Sonoma, CA
(707) 935-5073

Mid-Peninsula LSG
Linda Goffinet
Stanford, CA
(415) 493-6511

Plumas/Lassen County LDSG
Luana Phinney
Susanville, CA
(916) 257-7853

Lyme Disease Resource Center
Phyllis Mervine
Ukiah, CA
(707) 575-5133

Siskiyou LDA & Service Group
Susan Young
Ureka, CA
(916) 842-5003

Lyme Disease Support Group
Linda Nicola
Woodland Hills, CA
(818) 348-0932

COLORADO
Rocky Mountain LSG
Dietra DuPray
Denver, CO
(800) 886-9223

Rocky Mountain LD Network
Jan Derby
Englewood, CO
(303) 689-1299

CONNECTICUT
Bristol-Burlington LSG
Linda Dallon Gordon
Bristol, CT
(203) 589-2216

Easton LSG
Dolly Curtis
Easton, CT
(203) 372-4511

Greater Hartford LDSG
Kathleen Beaton, R.N.
East Hartford, CT
(203) 289-5811

Newton LDSG
Jay McMahan
Ridgefield, CT
(203) 438-5289

New Canaan LDSG
Cynthia Onorato
Ridgefield, CT
(203) 438-0682

Tri-State LSG
Diane Magnuson
Salisbury, CT
(203) 435-9914

FLORIDA
LSG of Gainesville
Gary and Virginia Smith
Gainesville, FL
(904) 373-7087

Fred Lawson
Leesburg, FL
(904) 360-2301

LSG of South Florida
Linda Carrizales
Miramar, FL
(305) 432-2234

Lyme Disease Survivors, Central
   Florida
Norma Shackleton
Ocala, FL
(904) 237-0345

GEORGIA
Georgia LD Network
Dot Welsh
(800) 456-LYME

IDAHO
Silver Valley LSG
Ramona Jones
Cataldo, ID
(208) 682-4087

ILLINOIS
St. Louis/Belleville Lyme Project
Diana Svec
Belleville, IL
(800) 756-5757

Quad Cities LD Information and
   SG
Joan Glaus
Coal Valley, IL
(309) 799-5500

LDSG of Southern Illinois
Susan Harryman
Marion, IL
(618) 997-7848

Central Illinois LSG
Bonnie Warfield and Alice
   Hunter
Tower Hill, IL
(217) 567-3345

INDIANA
Vanderburgh County LSG
Charlene Glover
Evansville, IN
(812) 471-1990

Central Indiana LSG
Theresa Parks
Indianapolis, IN
(317) 297-1695

Terre Haute LSG
Connie Lawrence
Terre Haute, IN
(812) 466-1469

KENTUCKY
Kentucky Lyme Support
   Network
(800) 666-0256

Candace Young
Independence, KY
(606) 283-1038

MARYLAND
Chesapeake Lyme Society
Pam Brenza
Annapolis, MD
(410) 757-0043

Donna Mauck
Darnestown, MD
(301) 869-2533

Maryland Lyme Support Group
Wendy P. Feaga, D.V.M.
Ellicott City, MD
(410) 531-6330

MASSACHUSETTS
Mid-Massachusetts LSG
Claire D'Andrea and Jill Vahey
Upton, MA
(508) 529-6316

Martha's Vineyard LD Action
   Committee
Patricia M. Arnold
Vineyard Haven, MA
(508) 693-4996
(June 15 through summer)

MICHIGAN
LDSG of Southeast Michigan
Meredith Spencer Foster
Ann Arbor, MI
(no number available)

Upper Peninsula Lyme Support
Paula Sten
Atlantic Mine, MI
(906) 482-5772

SE Michigan Support Group
Laurie Eichstead
Brighton, MI
(313) 231-9462

Thumb Area LSG
Jan Monson
Caro, MI
(517) 673-1586

Blue Water Area LDSG
Amelia Winkler and Pat Phipps
Croswell, MI
(313) 679-4843

Michigan Lyme Borreliosis SG
Jane Huegel
Saginaw, MI
(517) 792-7170

Mid-Michigan Lyme Network
Karen Norcross
St. Johns, MI
(517) 224-8340

MINNESOTA
We Care LDSG
Pearl Brennan
Austin, MN
(507) 433-6400

North Metro LDS Network
Carol Bolte
Columbia Heights, MN
(612) 574-0231

Duluth/Superior LDSG
Tom Grier
Duluth, MN
(218) 728-3914

Iron Range LDSG
Lois Anderson
Iron, MN
(218) 263-6021

St. Louis Park LDSG
Linda Hanner
Maple Plain, MN
(612) 972-3762

Princeton Arthritic and Lyme SG
Joyce Wenzel
Princeton, MN
(612) 389-4743

Wilmar LSG
Lynn Zimmer
Raymond, MN
(612) 967-4306

LD Coalition of Minnesota
Laura and Dan Sawyer
Roseville, MN
(612) 483-2464

MISSOURI
Lyme Disease Self-Help Group
Randy Morse
Cape Girardeau, MO
(314) 339-1980

Midwest Lyme Disease SG
Kathy Cavert
Independence, MO
(816) 252-6159

Gateway Lyme SG
Tony Calandro
St. Louis, MO
(800) 695-9949

NEBRASKA
Nebraska Lyme Association
Sarah Roemer
Lincoln, NE
(402) 488-7479

NEW JERSEY
Take Tyme for Lyme SG
Diana Haskell
Bayville, NJ
(908) 269-5764

Lyme Disease Network of NJ
Carol Stolow
East Brunswick, NJ
(908) 390-5027

New Jersey LDSG
Carol Gabriel
Freehold, NJ
(908) 462-9021

Lyme Disease Assn. No. NJ, Inc.
Hasbrouck Heights, NJ
Kim Uffleman (201) 391-4495
Sally Timpone (201) 288-5249

Lyme Disease Coalition of NJ
Peggi Sturmfels
Jackson, NJ
(908) 657-2190

LD Assoc. of Central Jersey
Kerry Fordyce
Governor's Advisory Council on
 LD
Ken Fordyce
Jackson, NJ
(908) 363-1980

Southern Ocean County
 Hospital
Margaret Janasie
Manahawkin, NJ
(609) 971-1848

Morris Area LSG
Elsie Anderson
Morristown, NJ
(201) 267-4251

Teen Lyme Line of No. Jersey
Chris Lang
Morristown, NJ
(201) 984-2860
(evenings)

LSG for Teens and Parents
Christine Hatfield
Neptune, NJ
(908) 922-8462

Med Center of Ocean County
 LG
Karen Fennesay
Point Pleasant, NJ
(908) 295-6389

South Jersey LSG
Nicki Giberson
Port Republic, NJ
(609) 652-0366

Lyme Disease SG of Northwest
  Jersey
Mary Ellen Monahan
Rockaway, NJ
(201) 625-0798

Mandy Memorial LDSG
Mary Schmidt
Sayreville, NJ
(908) 238-6405

LD Resource Group, South
  Jersey
Patricia Baker
Waterford Works, NJ
(609) 768-0888

Lyme Care Support Group
Judy DeBow
Wrightstown, NJ
(609) 758-9155

NEW MEXICO
Quantum Health Resources
Albuquerque, NM
(800) 224-3336

New Mexico Chapter LDSG
Helen Ingoglia
Rio Rancho, NM
(505) 891-8533

NEW YORK
Orange County LSG
Eileen Gould
Cornwall, NY
(914) 534-9957

New York State LD Coalition
Martha Kramer
Garrison, NY
(914) 424-4051

Abel Health
Ed Abel
Great Neck, NY
(800) 451-2235

Westchester LSG
Betty Gross
Irvington-on-Hudson, NY
(914) 591-7023

East End LSG
Mary Ann Tupper
Long Island, NY
(516) 283-5493

Lyme Borrelia Out-Reach
Stephen Nostrom
Mattituck, NY
(516) 298-9606

Lyme Disease SG of Middletown
Eileen Wright
Middletown, NY
(914) 343-4469

LSG of Rockland County
Edye Green
New City, NY
(914) 634-1588

LD Association of NY-
  Manhattan
Jessica Rose
New York, NY
(212) 472-5164

Long Island Lyme Association
Diane Leary
Plainview, NY
(516) 797-5963

So. Tier of Western NY LSG
Linda Chisholm
Portville, NY
(716) 933-6416

Northern Westchester LSG
Jill Branch
Purdy, NY
(914) 621-1602

Westchester Children's LSG
Barbara Goldklang, Pleasantville
(914) 769-6243
Pat Walsh, Scarsdale
(914) 472-3496

Mercy Community Hospital
  LSG
Carol Eckes
Sparrowbush, NY
(914) 856-2302

LD Association of NY–Staten
  Island
Joyce Mennella
Staten Island, NY
(718) 981-4570

Dr. Lloyd Miller, D.V.M.
  (resource)
Troy, NY
(518) 283-1166

OHIO
Ohio Lyme Support Network
(represents five LSGs)
(800) 666-0256

Warren County LSG
Linda Flory
Centerville, OH
(513) 885-7880

Midwest LD Referral Center
Craig Cleveland, M.D.
Cincinnati, OH
(513) 321-3776

Tri-State Lyme Vine SG
Lynda Van Hoene
Cincinnati, OH
(513) 561-5794

Greater Cleveland LSG
Ann Hirschberg
Cleveland, OH
(216) 235-4163

St. Clairsville, OH LS Groups
Cindy Jones and Judy Coleman
St. Clairsville, OH
(614) 695-1945

N.E. Ohio LDSG
Bernice Link
Thompson, OH
(216) 298-3446

Mahoning LSG
Marge Helle
Youngstown, OH
(216) 782-4528

OREGON
Springfield LDSG
McKenzie Willamette Hospital
Community Education Dept.
Springfield, OR
(503) 726-4459

PENNSYLVANIA
Beaver County LDSG
Anna Marie Smith
Beaver Falls, PA
(412) 846-1659

The Lyme Project SG
Neil Goldstein
Bry Athyn, PA
(215) 756-4022

Clearfield Area LSG
Linda Dixon
Clearfield, PA
(814) 756-4022

DuBois Area LDSG
Anne Posteraro
DuBois, PA
(814) 371-2747

LSG of Erie County
Deb Abbot
Erie, PA
(814) 866-3452

Mercer County LD Info. and SG
Ann Vesonder
Hermitage, PA
(412) 962-7553

Clarion Area LDSG
Brenda Fulton
Lucinda, PA
(814) 226-7322

Pittsburgh LDSG
Rene Landis
Pittsburgh, PA
(412) 963-9395

Western PA Lyme Information
Ronda Bartholomew
Sharon, PA
(412) 981-5728

North Central PA LDSG
Yolanda Wolfel
St. Mary's, PA
(814) 781-6332

Northwestern PA LSG
Dave and Sally Coates
Sugar Grove, PA
(814) 489-3898

LDSG of Huntingdon Valley
Dr. Barbara Caruso
Willow Grove, PA
(215) 657-8135

First Capital Lyme Network,
  S.E. PA
Rosemary Grove
Windsor, PA
(717) 246-9094

SOUTH CAROLINA
South Carolina LD Network
Don and Barbara Richardson
Columbia, SC
(800) 477-7040

TENNESSEE
Mid-South LDSG
Cheryl Leventhal
Memphis, TN
(901) 682-3188

Norris Blackburn (resource)
Morristown, TN
(615) 586-7071

TEXAS
Texas Lyme Chapter
Mamie Rich
Irving, TX
(214) 650-0066

Muleshoe Area LDSG
Sam Harlan
Muleshoe, TX
(806) 925-6687

VIRGINIA
Southwest VA and NE
  Tennessee LSG
Charlotte Caulkins
Bristol, VA
(703) 669-2798

Central VA LDSG
Patricia Arnold
Gordonsville, VA
(703) 832-3049

No. Virginia LDSG
Sally Rabenko
Herndon, VA
(703) 709-0890

LD Information Ctr. of VA
Joan McCallum
Oakton, VA
(703) 264-1264

Southwestern VA LDSG
Paula Pruett
Roanoke, VA
(703) 774-0257

WEST VIRGINIA
WV Lyme Support Network
(represents ten SGs in WV)
(800) 666-0256

WISCONSIN
Fox Valley LDSG
Beckie Murdock
Black Creek, WI
(414) 984-3213

St. Agnes Hospital LDSG
Kathryn Montgomery
Fond du Lac, WI
(414) 921-5588

Ironwood VP Lyme Support
Peg Sutherland
Gilo, WI
(715) 561-5534

Green Bay LSG
Lucie Schuler
Green Bay, WI
(414) 497-9161

Hudson LDSG
Pat Duncan
Hudson, WI
(715) 385-5454

Lyme Resource Group-Madison
Jeanette Wheat
Madison, WI
(608) 244-6425

Greater Milwaukee LSG
Jackie Tort
Milwaukee, WI
(414) 342-0400

LaCrosse LDSG
Leslie Zantow
Onalaska, WI
(608) 526-3629

Fox Valley LSG
Monica Johnson
Seymour, WI
(414) 833-6617

Superior LDSG
Rebecca Nelson
Superior, WI
(715) 392-8545

CANADA
Lyme Borreliosis SG of Ontario
John Scott
Fergus, Ontario
(519) 843-3646

Lyme Borreliosis SG
Philip Williams, M.D.
Ajax, Ontario
(416) 683-3372

FOUNDATIONS AND INDEPENDENT RESOURCES

AUTHOR'S NOTE: It is up to the individual to interview or otherwise screen these resources for his or her purposes.

American Lyme Disease Alliance
Joseph Burke, President
P.O. Box 230
Pitman, NJ 08071
(609) 863-8540

American Lyme Disease
    Foundation, Inc.
David Weld, Executive Director
Royal Executive Park
3 International Drive
Rye Brook, NY 10573
(914) 934-9155

Families USA
Ron Pollack, Executive Director
Phyllis Torda, Director of
    Health and Social Policy
1334 G Street, NW
Washington, DC 20005
(202) 628-3030

Lyme Awareness Productions
P.O. Box 1236
Pt. Pleasant Beach, NJ 08742
(908) 899-2642

Lyme Disease Foundation
Thomas Forschner, Executive
    Director
P.O. Box 462
Tolland, CT 06084-0462
(203) 871-2900

Lyme Disease Network
William Stolow, President
43 Winton Road
East Brunswick, NJ 08816
(908) 390-5027

Prevent Lyme Foundation, Inc.
Lynn Latchford, Executive
    Director
P.O. Box 758
Morristown, NJ 07963-0758
(201) 292-1909 (NJ residents)
(800) 479-9299

David Testone and Associates
Brewster, NY 10509
(914) 278-7813

VOICE (Victims of Insurance
    Company Exploitation)
Anne Ebert, Founding Director
Howell, NJ
(908) 370-2271

Appendix B:
Newsletters

Newsletters have varied subscription/mail charges for monthly to quarterly publications.

LymeAid
Kathy Cavert, Editor
P.O. Box 3135
Independence, MO 64055
(816) 252-6159

Lyme Disease Update
Charlene Glover, Owner/Editor
1511 Stockwell Road
Evansville, IN 47715
(812) 471-1990

Lyme Letter
Westchester Lyme Support
   Group
Betty Gross
P.O. Box 82
Irvington-on-Hudson, NY 10533
(914) 591-7023

Lymelight
John Anderson, Editor
Lyme Disease Foundation
P.O. Box 462
Tolland, CT 06084-0462
(203) 871-2900

Lyme Lines
National Institutes of Health
Laurie Doepel, Editor
Box AMS
9000 Rockville Pike
Bethesda, MD 20892

The Lyme Threat
American Lyme Disease Alliance
Joseph Burke, Editor
P.O. Box 230
Pitman, NJ 08701
(609) 863-8540

The Lyme Times
Lyme Disease Resource Center
Phyllis Mervine, Editor
P.O. Box 1423
Ukiah, CA 95482
(707) 575-5133

Lyme Treatment News
National Lyme Community
    Research Institute
Richard Lynch, Editor
17 Monroe Avenue
Staten Island, NY 10301
(718) 273-3740

the ticked-off tract
Ames to Please Publications
Laura Ames, Editor/Publisher
325 Fresno Street
Coalinga, CA 93210
(209) 935-0914

Lyme Disease Education Project
(patient/physician perspectives
    from the United States and
    Canada)
Lora Mermin, Editor
321 Palomino Lane
#2 South
Madison, WI 53705
(608) 231-2199

Bibliography

Alexander, Ames. "Profit Motive Alleged in Lyme Disease Care." *Asbury Park Press*, 29 March 1992.

"A Model Plan." *The Fresno Bee*, 5 September 1990.

Appel, Max J. G. "Lyme Disease in Dogs and Cats." In *The Compendium*. Ithaca, N.Y.: Cornell University, May 1990.

Asbrink, Eva, and Anders Hovmark. "Early and Late Cutaneous Manifestations in Ixodes-borne Borreliosis (Erythema Migrans Borreliosis, Lyme Borreliosis)." *Annals of the New York Academy of Sciences*, 1989.

Bakken, Lori L., et al. "Performance of 45 Laboratories Participating in a Proficiency Testing Program for Lyme Disease Serology." *Journal of the American Medical Association*, 19 August 1992, pp. 891–95.

Barrett, Katherine, and Richard Greene. "How to Get the Most from Your Health Insurance." *Ladies' Home Journal*, June 1992, p. 52.

Battelle, Phyllis. "My Doctor Said I Had AIDS—I Didn't." *Redbook*, March 1992.

Belkin, Lisa. "In Lessons on Empathy, Doctors Become Patients." *New York Times*, 4 June 1992.

Blackburn, Norris. "Lyme Disease: A Serious Threat." *Blue Ridge Outdoors*, October 1992, pp. 16–17.

Bleiweiss, John. "When to Suspect Lyme Disease." *The Lyme Threat*. American Lyme Disease Alliance, Fall 1992.

Bowen, G. Stephen, Terry L. Schulze, and William Parkin. "Lyme Disease in New Jersey, 1978–1982." *Yale Journal of Biology & Medicine* (1984):661–68.

Bozsik, Bela P., et al. "Combined Antibiotic Treatment of Lyme Borrel-iosis." Abstract 67, *V International Conference on Lyme Borreliosis.* Arlington, Va.: May 1992.

Brataas, Anne. "Living with Lyme Disease." *St. Paul Express*, 16 May 1992.

Brenner, Carl. "Lyme Disease: Asking the Right Questions." *Science* 257 (25 September 1992).

Brody, Jane. "Dealing with Lyme Disease Can Be a Tough Call." *New York Times*, 26 August 1992.

———. "For Time Outdoors, Ways to Avoid Lyme Disease." *New York Times*, 26 June 1991.

Bukro, Casey. "Lyme Disease Presents Threat to Woodlands Hikers, Campers." *Chicago Tribune*, 16 June 1991.

Burgdorfer, Willy. "Discovery of the Lyme Disease Spirochete: A His-torical Review." *International Journal of Microbiology and Hygiene*, Series A, Medical Microbiology, Infectious Diseases, Virology, Para-sitology (1986):7–9.

———. "Lyme Borreliosis: Ten Years After Discovery of the Etiologic Agent, *Borrelia burgdorferi*." *Infection*. Special reprint, vol. 19 (1991):3–7.

Burrascano, Joseph J., Jr. "Diagnostic Hints and Treatment Guidelines for Lyme Disease." October 1991. Pamphlet.

———. "Late Stage Lyme Disease: Treatment Options and Guide-lines." *Internal Medicine* 10 (December 1989).

———. "Lyme Disease Rehabilitation." Treatment paper guide-lines, presented at Lyme Disease Consensus Meeting, November 1992.

———. Letter. *Internal Medicine World Report*, 10 December 1991.

———. "Transmission of *Borrelia burgdorferi* by Blood Transfusion." Abstract 256A, *V International Conference on Lyme Borreliosis.* Arlington, Va.: May 1992.

Burstein, Edward. "Coping, or Not Coping, with Stress." *UC the Inde-pendent Press*, 8 January 1992, p. 11.

Cameron, Daniel J., and Victoria P. Malara. "Successful Retreatment of Lyme." Abstract 70C, *V International Conference on Lyme Bor-reliosis.* Arlington, Va.: May 1992.

Cartter, Matthew L., et al. "Epidemiology of Lyme Disease in Connecticut." *Connecticut Medicine*, June 1989, pp. 320–23.

Cassem, Edwin H. "When Symptoms Seem Groundless." *Emergency Medicine*, 15 June 1992, pp. 191–99.

Cavert, Kathy. "Surviving Lyme Disease." *LymeAid*, June/July 1992.

———. "Lyme Disease Questionnaire." Midwest Lyme Disease Association, November 1990.

Centers for Disease Control, Morbidity and Mortality Weekly Report. "Effectiveness in Disease and Injury Prevention: Lyme Disease Knowledge, Attitudes, and Behaviors—Connecticut, 1992." *Archives of Dermatology* 128 (September 1992):1171.

———. "Lyme Disease—United States." *Morbidity and Mortality Weekly Report*, 2 October 1992, pp. 726–27.

———. "Lyme Disease Surveillance Case Definition." Program for prevention and control of Lyme disease, 1992.

Clark, Jane R., et al. "Facial Paralysis in Lyme Disease." *Laryngoscope*, November 1985.

Classen, Norma. "Lyme Disease Easiest to Cure When Diagnosed, Treated in Early Stages." *University Chronicle*. St. Cloud State University, 24 March 1992.

Coyle, P. K. "Neurologic Lyme Disease." *Seminars in Neurology* 12 (September 1992):2–10.

Crist, Charles L. "Pulse Therapy with Antibiotic Needs More Research." *Lyme Disease Update*, November 1991.

Dattwyler, Raymond J. "Lyme Borreliosis: An Overview of the Clinical Manifestations." *Laboratory Medicine* 21 (May 1990):290–92.

Devery, Glenn. "Lyme Disease: A Tick(ing) Bomb." *Outdoor Life*, February 1988, p. 42.

Dinerman, Hal, and Allen Steere. "Lyme Disease Associated with Fibromyalgia." *Annals of Internal Medicine*, August 1992.

Doepel, Laurie K. "NIAID Scientists Develop Direct Method to Detect Presence of the Lyme Disease Spirochete." *Update*, April 1991.

Doepel, Laurie K., and Barbara Weldon. "Researchers Battle Lyme Disease." *Healthline*, June 1991.

Drulle, John. "Lyme Disease: Late Season Update." *Drug Therapy* 25 (August 1989):36–42.

————. "Pregnancy and Lyme Disease." *LymeAid*, August/September 1990.

Drummond, Roger. "Ticks and What You Can Do About Them." Berkeley, Calif.: Wilderness Press, 1990.

Durkin, Barbara J. "Spinal Tap Helps Doctor Spot Infection." *The Reporter Dispatch*, Westchester County, N.Y., 18 May 1992.

————. "New Way Found to Test for Lyme." *The Reporter Dispatch*, Westchester County, N.Y., 9 September 1992, p. 9.

Edelman, Robert. "Perspective on the Development of Vaccines Against Lyme Disease." *Vaccine* 9 (August 1991):531–32.

Ellis, B. J. "The Threat of Lyme Disease." *Columbia Metropolitan* 89 (July/August 1992):339–42.

Etling, Kathy. "Lyme Disease: What Makes It Tick." *Outdoor Life*, May 1990, p. 43.

Fallon, Brian A., et al. "The Neuropsychiatric Manifestations of Lyme Borreliosis." *Psychiatric Quarterly* 63 (Spring 1992):95–117.

Feaga, Wendy P. *Handbook on Lyme Borreliosis*. 4th ed. Ellicott City, Md., June 1991.

Fernandez, Ana, and Leonard Sigal. "Trends in the Therapy of Lyme Disease." *Today's Therapeutic Trends*. University of Medicine and Dentistry of NJ, Robert Wood Johnson Medical School, 1992.

Finn, Albert F., Jr., and Raymond J. Dattwyler. "The Immunology of Lyme Borreliosis." *Laboratory Medicine* 21 (May 1990):305.

Flach, Allan J., and Paul E. Lavoie. "Episcleritis, Conjunctivitis, and Keratitis As Ocular Manifestations of Lyme Disease." *Ophthalmology* 97 (August 1990):973–75.

Freedman, Mitchell. "Ticks Get No Shelter on Island." *Newsday*, 7 July 1991.

Friedman, Emily. "Insurers Under Fire." *HMQ*, Third Quarter 1991, p. 23.

Garcia-Monco, Juan C., et al. "*Borrelia burgdorferi* in the Central Nervous System: Experimental and Clinical Evidence for Early Invasion." *Journal of Infectious Disease*, June 1990, pp. 1187–93.

Georgilis, Kostis, M. Peacocke, and M. S. Klempner. "Fibroblasts Protect the Lyme Disease Spirochete, *Borrelia burgdorferi*, from Ceftriaxone in Vitro." *Journal of Infectious Disease*, August 1992, pp. 440–44.

Gerber, Michael A., et al. "Risk of Acquiring Lyme Disease or Babesiosis from a Blood Transfusion in Connecticut," Abstract 361, *V International Conference on Lyme Borreliosis*. Arlington, Va.: May 1992.

Gerber, Paul C. "How to Hold Third-Party Payers Accountable for Second-Guessing You." *Physician's Management*, December 1990, p. 23.

Gerlin, Andrea. "Lyme Disease Spurs Disputes over Treatment." *The Wall Street Journal*, 28 July 1992.

Hall, R. D., et al. "Research on Ticks and Tick-borne Pathogens in Missouri—An Interim Research Report." *Missouri Medicine* 89 (June 1991):339–42.

Hassler, Dieter, et al. "Pulsed High-Dose Cefotaxime Therapy in Refractory Lyme Borreliosis." Letter. *The Lancet* 338 (20 July 1991):193.

Hearn, Wayne. "Expert Witness Sued for Giving His Opinion During Peer Review." *American Medical News*, 11 May 1992, p. 3.

Heltzel, Jo Ann. *Learning About Lyme Disease*. Woodbury, Minn.: privately published, 1991.

Jaffe, Herb. "Blues File Suit Against Health Care Firms, MD and Others in $4 Million Bilk." *The Star Ledger*, Newark, N.J., 14 September 1992.

Johns, Stephanie. "Doctors' Favorite Doctors." *New Jersey Monthly*, April 1992, pp. 42–46.

Katzel, James H. "Is There a Consensus in Treatment of Lyme Borreliosis?" Paper presented at the Lyme Borreliosis Foundation International Symposium in California, April 1991.

———. "What Is the Best Treatment for Lyme Borreliosis (Lyme Disease)?" *the ticked-off tract*, October 1992.

———. "What Type of Doctor Treats Lyme Disease?" *the ticked-off tract*, November 1992.

Katzel, James H., and Ross I. Ritter. "Lyme Disease Without Erythema Migrans, Five Case Studies." Abstract 55C, *V International Conference on Lyme Borreliosis*. Arlington, Va.: May 1992.

Keller, Tracey L., J. J. Halperin, and M. Whitman. "PCR Detection of *Borrelia burgdorferi* DNA in Cerebrospinal Fluid of Lyme Neuroborreliosis Patients." *Neurology*, January 1992, pp. 32–34.

Khare, Madan L. "Lyme Disease Forum: Peril for Household Pets." *The Messenger-Press* (New Jersey), 25 July 1991.

Kong, Delores. "Swift Treatment Urged to Avert Lyme Disease." *The Boston Globe*, 20 August 1992.

Lavoie, Paul E. "Failure of Published Antibiotic Regimens in L. Borreliosis: Observations on Prolonged Oral Therapy." Paper presented at the Lyme Borreliosis International Conference, Sweden, 1990.

———. "Lyme Disease." *Conn's Current Therapy*. 1991.

———. "Lyme Disease: Pregnancy." *Rakel's Current Therapy*. 1991.

Leary, Warren E. "Exhibition Examines Scientists' Complicity in Nazi-Era Atrocities." *New York Times*, 10 November 1992, p. C3.

Liegner, Kenneth B., et al. "Culture-Confirmed Treatment Failure of Cefotaxim and Minocycline in a Case of Lyme Meningoencephalomyelitis in the United States." Abstract 63, *V International Conference on Lyme Borreliosis*. Arlington, Va.: May 1992.

———. "Recurrent Erythema Migrans Despite Extended Antibiotic Treatment with Minocycline in a Patient with Persisting BB Infection." *M. Dermatology*, August 1992.

Lissman, Barry A., et al. "Spirochete-Associated Arthritis (Lyme Disease) in a Dog." *Journal of the American Veterinary Association* 185 (15 July 1984):219–20.

Logigian, Eric, Richard F. Kaplan, and Allen Steere. "Chronic Neurologic Manifestations of Lyme Disease." *New England Journal of Medicine*, 22 November 1990, pp. 1438–44.

Luft, Benjamin J., et al. "Invasion of the Central Nervous System by *Borrelia burgdorferi* in Acute Disseminated Infection." *Journal of the American Medical Association*, 11 March 1992, pp. 1364–67.

"Lyme Disease: Not Just Deer Ticks." *American Health*, June 1989.

"Lyme Disease Clinic to Open." *Shoshone* (Idaho) *News Press*, 19 September 1990.

Lyme Disease Coalition of New Jersey, Inc. "Lyme Disease Patient Position Paper." 1992.

MacDonald, Alan B. "Gestational Lyme Borreliosis Implications for the

Fetus." *Rheumatic Disease Clinics of North America* 15, November 1989.

MacDonald, Alan B., J. L. Benach, and W. Burgdorfer. "Stillbirth Following Maternal Lyme Disease." *NY State Journal of Medicine*, 1987.

Magid, David, et al. "Prevention of Lyme Disease After Tick Bites: A Cost-Effective Analysis." *New England Journal of Medicine*, 20 August 1992.

Magnarelli, Louis A. "Derologic Diagnosis of Lyme Disease." *Annals, New York Academy of Sciences*, 1 May 1987.

Magnarelli, Louis A., et al. "Antibodies to *Borrelia burgdorferi* in Rodents in the Eastern and Southern United States." *Journal of Clinical Microbiology*, June 1992, pp. 1449–52.

Magnarelli, Louis, and John F. Anderson. "Ticks and Biting Insects Infected with the Etiologic Agent of Lyme Disease, *Borrelia burgdorferi*." *Journal of Clinical Microbiology*, August 1988, pp. 1482–86

Marconi, Richard T., W. Hauglum, and Claude F. Garon. "Species-specific Identification of and Distinction Between *Borrelia burgdorferi* Genome Groups by Using 16S RNA-Directed Oligonucleotide Probes." *Journal of Clinical Microbiology*, March 1992, pp. 628–32.

Marshall, Vincent. "Multiple Sclerosis Is a Chronic Central Nervous System Infection by a Spirochetal Agent." *Medical Hypotheses*. Animal Vaccine Laboratory, 1987.

Massarotti, Elena M., et al. "Treatment of Early Lyme Disease." *American Journal of Medicine*, April 1992, pp. 396–403.

Masters, Edwin J. "Erythema Migrans of Lyme Disease." *The Solution*. Special ed. 1992.

Masters, Edwin J., Pamela Lynxwiler, and Julie Rawlings. "Spirochetemia Two Weeks Post Cessation of Six Months Continuous P.O. Amoxicillin Therapy." Abstract 65, *V International Conference on Lyme Borreliosis*. Arlington, Va.: May 1992.

McCarthy, Laura Flynn. "Far from the Medical Mainstream." *Cosmopolitan*, June 1992, p. 263.

Mermin, Lora, ed. *Lyme Disease 1991: Patient/Physician Perspectives from the U.S. and Canada*. Madison, Wis.: The Lyme Disease Education Project, 1991.

Moran, Stephen J. "Physical, Financial Strain of Lyme Disease Addressed." *The Press of Atlantic City*, 15 November 1992.

Moulton, Chris. "Lyme Disease: New Facts Only Add to Diagnostic Frustrations." *Advance for Med Lab Professionals*, 29 July 1991, pp. 18–19.

Mueller, Mark. "Lyme Disease Infects State." *The Trentonian*, 23 December 1991.

National Institute of Allergy and Infectious Diseases. "Lyme Disease." *Backgrounder*, June 1991.

National Institutes of Health. "New NIH Research Grants on Lyme Disease." Department of Health and Human Services Fact Sheet, 23 July 1990.

NIH State-of-the-Art Conference. "Diagnosis and Treatment of Lyme Disease." *Clinical Courier* 9 (August 1991).

Pachner, Andrew R., and Andrea Itano. "*Borrelia burgdorferi* Infection of the Brain." *Neurology*, October 1990, pp. 1535–40.

Paparone, Philip W. "There Is No Standard Approach to Lyme Disease: Your Management Must Be Individualized." *Modern Medicine* 60 (September 1992):335–37.

Payer, Lynn. *Disease Mongers: How Doctors, Drug Companies, and Insurers Are Making You Feel Sick*. New York: John Wiley & Sons, 1992.

Pfister, H. W., et al. "Latent Lyme Neuroborreliosis: Presence of *Borrelia burgdorferi* in the Cerebrospinal Fluid Without Concurrent Inflammatory Signs." *Neurology* 39 (1989):1118–20.

Piesman, Joseph, et al. "Duration of Tick Attachment and *Borrelia burgdorferi* Transmission." *Journal of Clinical Microbiology*, March 1987, pp. 557–58.

Pietrucha, Dorothy M. "Many Difficult Problems for Children with Lyme." *Lyme Times, Newsletter of the LD Resource Center* 3 (Summer 1992).

———. "Neurologic Manifestations of Lyme Disease in Children." Paper presented at the National Lyme B. Scientific Symposium, March 1990.

———. "Neurologic Manifestations, Treatment for Youngsters." *The Messenger Press*, 22 August 1991.

"Pinning Down the Lyme Disease Antibody." *Science News* 137 (1990):156.

Plotkin, Stanley A., and Georges Peter. "Treatment of Lyme Borreliosis." *Pediatrics* 88 (July 1991):176–79.

Post, John E. "Lyme Disease in Large Animals." *Lyme Disease Update*, April 1991.

Preac-Mursic, V., et al. "Survival of *Borrelia burgdorferi* in Antibiotically Treated Patients with Lyme Borreliosis." *Infection* 5 (1989): 355–59.

Schoen, Robert T. "Treatment of Lyme Disease." *Connecticut Medicine* 53 (June 1989):335–37.

Schutzer, Steven E., et al. "Sequestration of Antibody to *Borrelia burgdorferi* in Immune Complexes in Seronegative Lyme Disease." *The Lancet* 335 (10 February 1990):312–15.

Seligmann, Jean, et al. "Lyme Disease: Tiny Tick, Big Worry." *Newsweek*, 22 May 1989.

Sigal, Leonard H. "Lyme Disease: Don't Let Its Disguises Fool You." *Internal Medicine* 13 (June 1992):24–33.

Steere, Allen C. "Distinguishing Lyme Disease from Its Look-Alikes." *Emergency Medicine*, 15 August 1992, pp. 28–44.

Sturmfels, Peg. "Lyme Disease Forum: Parents Must Become Teachers and Advocates." *The Messenger-Press* (New Jersey), 22 August 1991.

Sullivan, Patricia. "Health Insurers Limit Drugs for Lyme Disease." *The Star Ledger*, Newark, N.J., 22 March 1992.

3M Company. "Employees Are Urged to Be Aware of Lyme Disease." *The Stemwinder*, 10 April 1991.

Vanderhoof, Irwin T., and Karen M. B. Vanderhoof-Forschner. "Lyme Disease: The Cost to Society." Paper prepared as a funded project for the Lyme Disease Foundation and the Society of Actuaries, July 1992.

Watson, Linda. "Bringing Up Baby." *Homecare*, September 1992, p. 41.

Weldon, Barbara. "Dr. Steere Reports on Long-term Effects of Lyme on Children." *Lyme Times, Newsletter of the LD Resource Center*, Summer/Fall 1991, p. 15.

————. "Lyme Ticks Hitch Ride on Birds." *Healthline*, June 1991.

Wheat, Jeanette W. "What You Haven't Heard About Lyme Disease." *Wisconsin Pharmacist*, July 1991, pp. 16–18.

Whitlow, Joan. "Home Therapy Comes with Price Markups." *Newark Star Ledger*, 29 March 1992.

Wormser, Gary P. "Treatment of *Borrelia burgdorferi* Infection." *Laboratory Medicine* 21 (May 1990):316–21.

Wormser, Gary P., et al. "Use of a Novel Technique of Cutaneous Lavage for Diagnosis of Lyme Disease Associated with Erythema Migrans." *Journal of the American Medical Association*, 9 September 1992, pp. 1311–13.

Index